Post-Covid Transformations

This volume explores the implications of the COVID-19 pandemic for the sustainability of the present global political and economic system and the extent to which that system may as a result be undergoing transformation. Towards this aim, the contributing authors raise a number of key questions. First, what is likely to be the impact of the pandemic on the current global order based on neoliberal hyper-globalization? Second, what insights do earlier pandemics along with other interrelated crises such as those of climate, inequality, social reproduction and continued fallout of the global financial crisis offer for understanding the medium- to long-term implications of COVID-19? Third, to what extent might the COVID pandemic lead to progressive political transformations? Towards this latter goal, the contributors to this volume also offer a number of suggestions as to what a post-COVID-19 world might look like and how post-COVID transformations might be channelled in a direction more conducive towards social justice and equality.

The chapters in this book were originally published as a special issue of *Globalizations*.

Kevin Gray is Professor of International Relations at the University of Sussex, United Kingdom. His research interests relate to the political economy of development, with a regional focus on East Asia. He has researched widely on the region, and in particular, on the political economy of both North and South Korea. He also has interests in Gramscian approaches to international relations and in theories of late development and state formation.

Barry Gills is Editor in Chief of *Globalizations* and Professor of Global Development Studies at the University of Helsinki, Finland. He has written widely on World System theory, neoliberalism, globalization, global crises, democracy, resistance, and transformative praxis.

Rethinking Globalizations

Edited by **Barry K. Gills**, *University of Helsinki, Finland* and **Kevin Gray**, *University of Sussex, UK.*

This series is designed to break new ground in the literature on globalization and its academic and popular understanding Rather than perpetuating or simply reacting to the economic understanding of globalization, this series seeks to capture the term and broaden its meaning to encompass a wide range of issues and disciplines and convey a sense of alternative possibilities for the future.

Labour Conflicts in the Global South
Edited by Andreas Bieler and Jörg Nowak

Time, Climate Change, Global Racial Capitalism and Decolonial Planetary Ecologies
Edited by Anna M. Agathangelou and Kyle D. Killian

Globalizations from Below
The Normative Power of the World Social Forum, Ant Traders, Chinese Migrants, and Levantine Cosmopolitanism
Theodor Tudoroiu

Economics and Climate Emergency
Edited by Barry K. Gills and Jamie Morgan

Global Political Leadership
In Search of Synergy
Małgorzata Zachara-Szymańska

Post-Covid Transformations
Edited by Kevin Gray and Barry Gills

The Reconfiguration of Twenty-first Century Latin American Regionalism
Actors, Processes, Contradictions and Prospects
Edited by Rowan Lubbock and Ernesto Vivares

For more information about this series, please visit:
https://www.routledge.com/Rethinking-Globalizations/book-series/RG

Post-Covid Transformations

Edited by
Kevin Gray and Barry Gills

Routledge
Taylor & Francis Group

LONDON AND NEW YORK

First published 2023
by Routledge
4 Park Square, Milton Park, Abingdon, Oxon OX14 4RN

and by Routledge
605 Third Avenue, New York, NY 10158

Routledge is an imprint of the Taylor & Francis Group, an informa business

Introduction, Chapters 1–5 and 7–10 © 2023 Taylor & Francis
Chapter 6 © 2021 Yanqiu Rachel Zhou. Originally published as Open Access.

British Library Cataloguing in Publication Data
A catalogue record for this book is available from the British Library

ISBN13: 978-1-032-36207-6 (hbk)
ISBN13: 978-1-032-36209-0 (pbk)
ISBN13: 978-1-003-33075-2 (ebk)

DOI: 10.4324/9781003330752

Typeset in Minion Pro
by Newgen Publishing UK

Publisher's Note
The publisher accepts responsibility for any inconsistencies that may have arisen during the conversion of this book from journal articles to book chapters, namely the inclusion of journal terminology.

Disclaimer
Every effort has been made to contact copyright holders for their permission to reprint material in this book. The publishers would be grateful to hear from any copyright holder who is not here acknowledged and will undertake to rectify any errors or omissions in future editions of this book.

Contents

Citation Information

The chapters in this book were originally published in the journal *Globalizations*, volume 19, issue 3 (2022). When citing this material, please use the original page numbering for each article, as follows:

For any permission–related enquiries please visit:
www.tandfonline.com/page/help/permissions

Notes on Contributors

Robert A. Denemark studies the history and evolution of the global system, and the ability of theories of world politics to apprehend that long-term view. He is professor of Global Politics in the Department of Political Science at the University of Delaware, USA. Given the pandemic, he is spending his 2020–2021 sabbatical as 'Virtual Visiting Scholar' at the Arrighi Center for Global Studies at Johns Hopkins University, USA.

Barry Gills is Editor in Chief of *Globalizations* and Professor of Global Development Studies at the University of Helsinki, Finland. He has written widely on World System theory, neoliberalism, globalization, global crises, democracy, resistance and transformative praxis.

Kevin Gray is Professor of International Relations at the University of Sussex, United Kingdom. His research interests relate to the political economy of development, with a regional focus on East Asia. He has researched widely on the region, and in particular, on the political economy of both North and South Korea. He also has interests in Gramscian approaches to international relations and in theories of late development and state formation.

Ryan Gunderson is an assistant professor of Sociology and Social Justice Studies in the Department of Sociology and Gerontology at Miami University, USA. His current research projects concern the potential effectiveness of proposed solutions to environmental problems; the social dimensions and environmental impacts of technology; and the renewal of classical and mid-twentieth century sociological theory.

Paul James is Professor of Globalization and Cultural Diversity in the Institute for Culture and Society at the Western Sydney University, Australia. He is author/editor of over 30 books, including *Globalization Matters* (with Manfred Steger; 2019) and *Urban Sustainability in Theory and Practice* (2015).

Habibul Haque Khondker is a professor of Social Sciences at Zayed University, Abu Dhabi, UAE. His most recent work is *Covid-19 and Governance* (Routledge 2021) co-edited with Jan Nederveen Pieterse and Haeran Lim.

Krishen Mehta is a former partner of PwC and currently serves as a Director of Tax Justice Network. He is Senior Global Justice Fellow at Yale University, USA, and a member of the steering group of the Independent Commission for Reform of International Corporate Taxation (ICRICT). Mehta is co-editor of *Global Tax Fairness* (2016) and *Tax Justice and Global Inequality* (2020).

James H. Mittelman is Distinguished Research Professor and University Professor Emeritus at the School of International Service, American University, USA. He is also Honorary Fellow at the Helsinki Collegium for Advanced Studies. He is the recipient of the International Studies

Association's 2010 Distinguished Scholar award in International Political Economy. Currently, he is writing a book on *Transformations in Capitalism.*

Alf Gunvald Nilsen is Professor of sociology at the University of Pretoria, South Africa. His research focuses on social movements and the political economy of development and democracy in the Global South. His most recent book is *Adivasis and the State: Subalternity and Citizenship in India's Bhil Heartland* (2018).

Brian Petersen is an associate professor in the Department of Geography, Planning and Recreation at Northern Arizona University, USA. His research and published work focus on climate change adaptation and landscape level conservation. His work draws on both social and natural science perspectives to interrogate contemporary natural resource and environmental challenges.

Thomas Pogge, having received his PhD in philosophy from Harvard, is Leitner Professor of Philosophy and International Affairs and founding Director of the Global Justice Program at Yale University, USA. He co-founded Academics Stand Against Poverty, an international network aiming to enhance the impact of scholars, teachers and students on global poverty, and Incentives for Global Health, which is a team effort toward creating new incentives to improve access to advanced pharmaceuticals worldwide.

Kwang-Yeong Shin is CAU-Fellow at the Department of Sociology, Chung-Ang University, South Korea. He has been doing research on the work, inequality, and welfare in East Asia. His most recent book is *Precarious Asia: Global Capitalism and Work in Japan, South Korea, and Indonesia* (co-authored by Arne L. Kalleberg and Kevin Hewison; 2021).

Manfred B. Steger is Professor of Sociology at the University of Hawai'i-Manoa, USA and Global Professorial Fellow at the Institute of Culture and Society, Western Sydney University, Australia. He is the author of twenty-eight books on globalization and social theory, including, *The Rise of the Global Imaginary: Political Ideologies from the French Revolution to the Global War on Terror* (2008) and *Globalization Matters: Engaging the Global in Unsettled Times* (with Paul James; 2019).

Diana Stuart is Associate Professor in the Sustainable Communities Program in the School of Earth Sciences and Environmental Sustainability at Northern Arizona University, USA. Her research examines environmental and social issues in industrial agriculture and how to transition to a more sustainable food system. Her work has explored ways to increase wild biodiversity, reduce fertilizer pollution and greenhouse gas emissions and support animal welfare.

Silke Trommer is Senior Lecturer in the Department of Politics at the University of Manchester, UK. Together with Dr Adrienne Roberts, Politics, University of Manchester, and Dr Erin Hannah, King's University College at Western University, she holds a Social Sciences and Humanities Research Council of Canada (SSHRC) Insight Development grant titled "*She Trades: Gendering Global Trade Governance*". The purpose of this research is to explore how and why the idea of addressing the gender-differential impact of trade is currently becoming a global policy norm.

Yanqiu Rachel Zhou is a professor in the Department of Health, Aging & Society and the Institute on Globalization and the Human Condition at McMaster University, Canada. She is the lead editor of *Sexualities, Transnationalism, and Globalization: New Perspectives* (published by Routledge, 2021) and a themed symposium on Transnationalism, Sexuality, and HIV Risk (published in Culture, Health & Sexuality, 2017), and the co-editor of two books (published by Routledge, 2016 and 2017) and a special issue of the journal, *Globalizations* on *Time and Globalization*, 2016.

Introduction: post-COVID transformations

Kevin Gray and Barry Gills

ABSTRACT
This article provides an introduction to the special issue on post-COVID transformations. We raise three sets of questions relating to the implications of the pandemic for the sustainability of the present global political and economic system and the extent to which that system may as a result be undergoing transformation. First, what is likely to be the impact of the pandemic on the current global order based on neoliberal hyperglobalization? Second, what insights do earlier pandemics along with other inter-related crises such as those of climate, inequality, social reproduction, and continued fallout of the global financial crisis offer for understanding the medium- to long-term implications of COVID-19. Finally, the special issue seeks to address the question of the extent to which the COVID pandemic may lead to progressive political transformations. We conclude with a summary of each of the individual contributions to this special issue.

The COVID-19 pandemic, that rapidly spread across the globe in the early months of 2020, has been nothing short of a colossal human tragedy. The World Health Organization has reported that by February 2022, 5.7 million people had died worldwide as a direct result of the disease (though the real figure may be higher).[1] Many millions more are likely to have suffered or are still suffering from the long-term effects of COVID. Beyond these direct medical impacts, countless livelihoods have been damaged or destroyed by the economic fallout of the pandemic, as well as by the restrictive measures adopted by governments to try and slow or halt its spread.

The pandemic has, as a result, raised urgent questions about the sustainability of the present global political and economic system. The global pandemic also raises important questions about what kinds of broader social, economic, political, and cultural transformations may be likely or possible in a post-COVID world. It is not yet clear whether such transformations will ultimately take a predominantly progressive or regressive character, though as the words projected onto a Santiago apartment building in the early days of Chile's first lockdown read, 'No volveremos a la normalidad porque la normalidad era el problema' (*we will not return to normal because normal was the problem*).

Indeed, what quickly became clear as the virus spread across the globe in early 2020 was that the pandemic was intimately related with pre-existing crisis tendencies, including increasing inequality, ecological breakdown, and climate change, that have facilitated COVID-19's emergence, enabled its rapid spread, and amplified its disastrous impacts on global public health. Understanding how these multiple global crises intersect and amplify each other is crucial for a critical understanding of possible post-COVID transformations and how political praxis could steer social transformations in a progressive direction.

Perhaps the greatest indictment of the pre-COVID 'normality' is how the impacts of the pandemic have not been experienced equally but rather have been profoundly shaped by and in turn further entrenched existing patterns of global inequality. Such patterns of inequality have manifested themselves both within and between countries. In the Global North, governments were relatively well placed to support stay-at-home quarantine orders and buffer the fallout of economic contraction with various forms of financial assistance, including existing social welfare schemes, support for paid furlough, and one-off financial assistance cheques.[2] In parts of the developing world, however, densely populated cities, inadequate public health infrastructures, greater vulnerability to slowdowns in demand for key exports and in tourism, all imposed a heavy toll on already marginalized populations. Furthermore, measures such as lockdowns that in wealthier countries proved valuable in buying time were much less effective in a number of developing countries, which were typically unable to buy up vital medical equipment such as ventilators and testing kits (Kahl & Wright, 2021, p. 213).

The pandemic has also deepened inequalities within individual countries. The well-off were typically able to keep their well-paid jobs and benefit from rising stock market values and house prices, while lower-paid workers were more likely to have jobs in sectors badly hit by the pandemic, such as tourism and hospitality, or had jobs with higher risks of exposure and lived in crowded accommodation.[3] This deepening inequality and vulnerabilization served to exacerbate ongoing trends towards right-wing populist politics and authoritarianism (Cooper, 2021). As Freedom House has pointed out, since the pandemic began, democracy and human rights have deteriorated in 80 countries, as various governments responded to the virus by engaging in abuses of power, the repression and silencing of critics, and the weakening of key institutions, often with the effect of undermining the very systems of accountability needed to protect public health.[4]

As we enter into the third year of the COVID-19 global pandemic, it is an appropriate juncture at which to take stock and assess what impact the pandemic is likely to have in the medium to longer term. In many respects, however, the full implications of the COVID-19 pandemic may not be revealed for many years to come. But as the contributions to this special issue suggest, certain patterns can already be identified. The contributors to this special issue, therefore, seek to raise a number of inter-related questions.

First, what is likely to be the impact of the pandemic on the current global order based on relentless neoliberal hyperglobalization? For at least the last four decades, the international economic system has been based on hegemonic norms of market-led development and pursuit of relentless commodification of labour, society, and nature, overseen in theory at least by a minimal night-watchman state. In many respects, however, hyperglobalization can be identified as a key contributor to the emergence of the pandemic. Global Extractivism of resources, with its attendant ecological and social destructiveness (see forthcoming *Special Forum on Global Extractivism and Alternatives in the Journal of Peasant Studies*, guest edited by Barry Gills, Markus Kröger, and Anja Nygren, 2022) has accelerated significantly during the Era of neoliberal globalization. This link between global economic activity and disease should not be surprising. As Mike Davies has argued, multinational capital has historically been a key driver of disease evolution, through the burning or logging of tropical forests, proliferation of factory farming, the explosive growth of slums, and informal employment. The elimination of the barriers between human populations and virus-carrying birds, bats, and mammals along with the emergence of factory farms and giant feedlots act as incubators of novel viruses (Davis, 2020, p. 17).

Efforts (or lack of them) by national governments to tackle the pandemic have also brought into question neoliberal norms surrounding the 'proper' role of the state in the economy, and in particular, the question of state capacity and its role in crisis management. Indeed, it is a paradox that in 2019, the Global Health Security Index listed both the United States and the United Kingdom as the two countries with the highest level of pandemic preparedness, whereas South Korea was placed 9th, while China was placed 51st.[5] Yet, the United States has seen 2766 deaths per million, and the United Kingdom 2370 deaths. In South Korea, on the other hand, it has been 134 per million and in China only 3.5.[6] The previous 'common sense' concerning the presumed superior capability of major states in the global north versus the global south was turned upside down by the actual course of the pandemic across the globe.

State capacity plays a key role in explaining these divergences. It has been argued, for example, that the United Kingdom's response to the pandemic was hindered by the regulatory state's bloated bureaucracy and the National Health Service's inability to procure medical supplies as just-in-time arrangements with overseas suppliers quickly broke down as a result of their vulnerability to global supply disruptions (Jones & Hameiri, 2021). Countries still possessing considerable state capacity, such as South Korea, on the other hand, were able to tackle early outbreaks while avoiding lockdown, while domestic pharmaceutical companies in close partnership with the state were able to manufacture medical supplies as well as export them to developed countries amidst global shortages (Kumar, 2021).

The pandemic has therefore brought into question the role of the state in the economy and whether we have witnessed the beginning of the end of (hyper) neoliberalism. As Apeldoorn and de Graaff point out, however, the binary logic of the retreat/return of the state potentially neglects the fact that the reconfiguration of the role of the state does not necessarily imply a fundamental break with global marketization or the end of neoliberalism (2022, p. 16). The potential fetishization of state capacity may also have profoundly regressive implications, as states deemed as having 'performed well' have also shifted the costs of tackling the pandemic on to the poor and vulnerable.

Relatedly, what role do the institutions of global governance have in pandemic management and global health more broadly, and how should such institutions be reformed in a post-COVID world? Tensions between the Trump administration and the World Health Organization in the early days of the pandemic were testament to how international cooperation can easily fall victim to geopolitical competition when perceived 'national interests' are at stake. Even more insidious, however, has been the aggressive resort to vaccine nationalism, whereby wealthy nations secured billions of doses of vaccines – enough to inoculate their citizens many times over – leaving citizens of poorer countries largely unvaccinated and leaving the world vulnerable to new variants emerging in unvaccinated populations. Indeed, former UK Prime Minister Gordon Brown has described this stockpiling of vaccines as 'one of the greatest policy failures of our times'.[7] While programmes such as COVAX were devised in order to deal with such problems, they have been seriously underfunded. Issues have similarly been raised around the question of intellectual property rights waivers and their role in getting life-saving medicines to the world's poorest peoples (Sariola, 2021). Such waivers have, perhaps not surprisingly, been opposed by the major pharmaceutical companies but they have also been opposed by leading Western governments.

The second question is to examine what insights earlier pandemics along with other inter-related crises can shed on potential post-COVID transformations. It has been widely noted, for example, that previous pandemics such as the Black Death and the 1918 'Spanish' flu brought about widespread societal transformations in their wake. There are instructive differences, however, not least the rapidity of the development of vaccines that have saved countless lives and reduced the potential death toll of COVID-19. Other crises, such as the 2007–2008 global financial crisis (GFC) and the ongoing climate emergency, also provide valuable lessons as to the likelihood or otherwise of meaningful societal transformations. Indeed, many of the questions raised above concerning the fate of neoliberal hyperglobalization were also raised in the aftermath of the 2007–2008 global financial crisis, and thus, there are lessons here for judging the potential for reforms that may help prevent the emergence of the next pandemic and the mitigation of its impact on public health. In addition, the climate crisis is a particularly important comparative case, not least due to the direct interconnections between the two, but also in terms of shedding light on how crises are addressed or otherwise.

Finally, perhaps most importantly, the special issue seeks to address the question of the extent to which the COVID pandemic may lead to progressive political transformations. The pandemic has to date led to a wide range of diverse forms of social mobilization and protest, thereby ' … revealing the nature of the COVID-19 emergency as a moment of political suspension and heightened social confrontation' (Gerbaudo, 2020). In March 2021, The Economist reported that COVID-related protests had taken place in 86 countries since the start of the pandemic, and were typically driven by economic hardship, psychological exhaustion, and scepticism about governments' handling of the crisis.[8] The Black Lives Matter protests in the early summer of 2020, for example, were a response to police violence in the United States, but were also intimately related to how COVID-19 served to exacerbate underlying problems of racial injustice, isolation, frustration, and stagnation, and resulting higher unemployment.[9] Many mobilizations have also had regressive aspects, however. Although anti-lockdown protests have been driven by class-based grievances relating to economic hardship, they have also frequently been associated with right-wing and anti-vaccine conspiracy theories that look unlikely to form the basis of a post-COVID progressive politics. Indeed, a sober analysis of the current juncture suggests that tendencies towards an increasingly regressive world order appear to be more dominant at the moment: e.g. increasing global inequality, the deepening of nationalist populism and authoritarianism, the weakening of global health governance, continued economic fallout from the pandemic, the subordination of urgent climate change mitigation measures to the imperative of restoring capitalist growth, and further degradation of individual freedoms and life chances. In contrast, however, in many countries and communities across the globe, mutual aid societies came into action, offering vital help and support to others more vulnerable or suffering from the effects of the pandemic on their own life and livelihood. The widespread acts of mutual support that emerged from people themselves give testimonial to the potential for severe crisis to generate not only acts of resistance, but also acts of positive and progressive transformation.

Summary of the papers

Robert Denemark (2022) argues in his contribution to this special issue that pandemics have been a recurrent phenomenon, although as with COVID-19, their impacts upon states have been highly differentiated. States endowed with the capacity to provide public sanitation, enforce quarantines, and take preventative medical action tend to grow in strength, while those in decline and with poor and corrupt leaderships are likely to enter into a vicious cycle whereby those characteristics are reinforced by their failure to deal effectively with pandemics. Pandemics have also had a significant impact on the cycle of class conflict. Population decline can strengthen labour's position and lead to wage increases, although labour shortages can ultimately lead to new methods of labour control, while alterations in labour and climatic conditions affect the possibility of future pandemics. Pandemics can lead to scapegoating along both class and ethnic lines, reflecting the fact that populations are not impacted by pandemics evenly, which can generate suspicion and resentment. Pandemics have a close relationship to broader global political change. Military victory and defeat can depend greatly on the dynamics of particular pandemics, with disease strongly shaping the fate of established empires and the rise of colonial expansion. As Denemark argues, many of these dynamics are discernible in the current crisis, even if their precise form has taken novel manifestations. As noted, the differential impact of COVID-19 can be seen in those countries which have still retained a considerable degree of state capacity compared with those that have largely been hollowed out. While the pandemic has not led to the high death rates as seen in the Black Death and the subsequent decline of feudalism, there is little doubt that COVID-19 has led to an intensification of class conflict. Furthermore, ethnic scapegoating has been prevalent with suspicion and prejudice in the West directed towards those of Asian ancestry. The pandemic has also intensified US–China tensions, leading not just to vaccine nationalism but potentially to new forms of alliances or international community between countries that have opted for Chinese and Russian vaccines. Denemark's contribution also includes a brief appendix that considers challenges in the way we see disease and offers some quick and useful technical information.

In her contribution, Silke Trommer (2022) examines the impact of the pandemic on global trade and health, along with their relationship to the global productive and reproductive economy. She argues that the pandemic has exacerbated socio-economic inequalities and insecurities amidst a broader crisis in social reproduction. In particular, the sharp decline in global trade has impacted upon supplies that are essential for social reproduction, such as drugs and medical equipment. The pandemic has also contributed towards the pushing of care work out of the productive economy into domestic settings. In terms of the impact of the pandemic on global trade governance, COVID-19 has led to a renewed debate about intellectual property (IP) rights for medicines and the efficacy of the World Trade Organization's (WTO) Agreement on Trade-Related Aspects of Intellectual Property Rights (TRIPS) mechanism. While the TRIPS waiver proposed by the Biden administration in response to COVID-19 has met considerable resistance, Trommer argues that in any case, it fails to address broader issues surrounding the global distribution of medicines. In addition, the global IP regime anchored in trade agreements is just one aspect of a wider set of policies through which corporations rather than states govern global production networks. Legal provisions in trade agreements create health and social reproductive inequalities by benefitting corporations providing healthcare products and services. They do this through curtailing government intervention and spending in health and other areas relevant for social reproduction. Indeed, the COVID-19 era has seen no slowdown in the reaching of such trade agreements. Trade policy circles have failed to respond to the pandemic with a meaningful overhaul of global trade relations, and there has been no ideational shift whereby trade is understood as a tool for equitable and sustainable forms of social reproduction. This thereby leaves the exploitative nature of global trade relations and their ambivalent relationship with public health and social reproduction largely intact.

As noted, the COVID-19 pandemic is closely inter-connected with other crises such as the climate emergency and the GFC. Diana Stuart, Brian Petersen, and Ryan Gunderson (2022) argue that there are strong parallels between the failure of many states to adopt effective responses to the COVID-19 pandemic and failures to tackle climate change. Indeed, these failures are related given that the pandemic and the climate crisis can both be traced to the manner whereby the economic growth imperative has led to the transformation in the relationship between humans and nature. Focusing on the United States, Stuart et al. argue that these failures rest on denialism, individualism, and techno-optimism. Climate change denial takes explicit forms, such as outright rejection that anthropogenic climate change exists and scepticism towards the scientific basis of claims that climate mitigation efforts are necessary and justifiable. The earlier stages of the COVID-19 pandemic saw the Chinese government suppress information about the outbreak, while US President Donald Trump downplayed and minimized the crisis, spread misinformation, and even withheld the resources needed for testing. The common thread here is the strong resistance to measures that might negatively impact economic growth. Yet the failure to tackle the climate or COVID-19 crisis can take implicit forms, such as the promotion of individualism as pretence for collective inaction. With regards to climate change, there is an emphasis on such individual adjustments as veganism or flying less, which fall vastly short of what is required to make a significant reduction in global emissions. With regard to COVID 19, the Trump administration left individual state governors to tackle the crisis, which led to a wide disparity between liberal and conservative states in terms of the types and effectiveness of the measures deployed. Both crises saw the prevalence of techno-optimism as a shared pretence for collective inaction. With regard to climate change, this included focusing on alternative energy sources and improvements in efficiency to address climate change, despite the fact that such solutions are likely to be insufficient. COVID-19 similarly saw a heavy emphasis on vaccines as a silver bullet capable of avoiding significant alternatives, social changes, and economic downturn. The common thread here is that these justifications serve to maintain the status quo and benefit the wealthy few.

In terms of charting future trajectories, Paul James and Manfred Steger (2022) argue that the pandemic is likely to lead to two outcomes. The first is an intensification of what the authors refer to as the 'great unsettling', namely a set of complex social dynamics of instability and volatility that refers to the massive destabilization dynamics that have led to a reconstitution of the ecological, economic, and political life on this planet. The second is the growing prevalence of disembodied relations, namely those relations mediated by codes and signs such as digital technology, which are overlaying and remaking the more embodied and material processes of global integration and interchange, thereby transforming the human planetary condition. This argument is put forward through a comparison of COVID-19 with the GFC. Both crises demonstrate the disjuncture between embodied placement and abstracted relations. On the one hand, the sub-prime housing boom that preceded the GFC was strongly rooted in particular localities. Each act of buying a home in a local neighbourhood continued to be enacted at the level of embodied placement, e.g. in specific American cities. Yet the loans were lifted out of embodied placement and linked to global sub-prime mortgage financing as part of a disembodied process that had been underway for a couple of decades, through such mechanisms as residential mortgage-backed securities, collateralized debt obligations, and credit default swaps. The COVID-19 pandemic on the other hand was widely assumed to have its origins in Wuhan's 'wet markets', if not as the source of the pandemic, then at least as a place of its initial spreading. Yet the embodied placement of disease transmission transformed into the more abstract national and global realm as fixed points in a matrix of epidemiological statistics.

James Mittelman (2022) deploys Fernand Braudel's schematic of three speeds of time, namely the immediate moment, the medium term of a decade or decades, and the longue durée. He argues that these speeds of time correspond to overlapping periods of vaccine nationalism, viral globalization, and runaway capitalism. In the immediate moment, Mittelman points to the role of vaccine nationalism, noting that vaccination has been seen simply as a biomedical challenge of producing a successful vaccine rather than a more comprehensive trifecta of science, politics, and profit. Without focusing on human behaviour, it is impossible to understand the failure of political leaders to prepare for a potential pandemic despite numerous warnings, along with the role of philanthropists and their motivations that go beyond simple altruism towards capital accumulation. In the medium term, Mittelman draws attention to viral globalization, in which questions are raised about the availability, access, and affordability of vaccines more generally, and the extreme inequality in distribution amidst ongoing tensions between a planetary health crisis and vaccine nationalism. In the longue durée, Mittelman sees a post-pandemic age characterized by runaway capitalism in which there are both continuities and discontinuities with prior forms of capitalism. Runaway capitalism is characterized by three integrally connected forms: algorithmic capitalism driven by digital innovations, cognitive capitalism wherein the knowledge portion of commodities outstrips the physical components that produce them, and philanthropic capitalism, which is a market-based for-profit approach to solving intractable problems such as poverty and environmental degradation.

In her contribution, Rachel Zhou (2022) picks up these themes in examining how vaccine nationalism has exposed the dangers of nationalist responses to the global pandemic. In the first instance, the COVID-19 pandemic has emerged in the context of a broader crisis of globalization including the GFC, increased tendencies towards nationalism and populism, and growing US–China rivalry. Within this context, Zhou goes on to examine the emergence of vaccine nationalism and its impact on poorer countries, including the extent to which COVID-19 has become a zero-sum geopolitical power game alongside a weakening of the WTO and global health governance more broadly. The COVAX facility has been under-resourced and its effectiveness has been undermined by unequal participation. Its funding mechanism heavily favours pharmaceutical corporations through providing them with a win–win situation regardless of whether their vaccines gain regulatory approval, and its reliance on philanthropic funding suggests vulnerability to donor fatigue. COVAX is an example of increased reliance on public–private partnerships, showing that private solutions and interests are privileged over public approaches. Vaccine nationalism thus represents a serious threat to global public health. Lack of timely access to vaccines in many lower-income countries may prolong the global threat of COVID-19, while short-term nationalist responses to the pandemic may lead to the re-naturalization of the nation-state, and the undermining of collective capacities in dealing with other impending global crises. As such, the coexistence of nationalist and globalist approaches to COVID-19 vaccines suggests simultaneous and contentious processes of globalization and deglobalization.

Both Alf Gunvald Nilsen (2022) and Kwang-Yeong Shin (2022) provide detailed case studies of how the COVID-19 pandemic has impacted upon India and South Korea, respectively. As Nilsen argues, the pandemic was initially downplayed by the Narendra Modi government and there were inadequate attempts to strengthen the resilience of the country's health sector. This was followed, however, by one of the world's strictest lockdowns. The severity of India's COVID-19 crisis was shaped by two pre-existing crises, namely that of social reproduction and the subsistence of the working poor, along with a crisis of India's secular and constitutional democracy. This disjuncture between the harsh lockdown and the minimal efforts made at strengthening the country's medical infrastructure owed much to the 'centrality of spectacle' in the political modus operandi of Modi and the Bharatiya Janata Party, which, as with the demonetization debacle in 2016, served to bolster Modi's strongman image and the loyalty of his support base while delivering little else. As Nilsen argues, the lockdown had a devastating impact on the working poor, a process that Nilsen refers to as 'social murder'. Relief and economic stimulus from the government were limited, even compared to India's poorer South Asian neighbours. The Modi government even used the crisis to push through further neoliberal reforms, both in the agricultural sector and with regards to new restrictive labour laws, thereby using the crisis as a mechanism for strengthening the machinery for social murder. The crisis has also coincided with a strengthening of hegemonic authoritarian populism, involving a scapegoating of Muslims, often through hate speech and vigilante violence, as well as through repression of political dissidents (activists, public intellectuals, lawyers, journalists) who have challenged the government's claims to be acting in the interests of the people.

As noted above, one country frequently praised for its effective response to containing the virus, is South Korea. However, as Shin (2022) argues, this seemingly positive response rests on negative social trends involving an increase in precarious labour and a deepening of social inequality. As with India, the crisis served to exacerbate pre-existing crisis tendencies within the South Korean economy, namely the segmented labour market based on firm size, gender, employment status, and inadequate social production. Indeed, the abrupt economic slowdown revealed the precarity of informal work, including the self-employed and other atypical workers. The pandemic accelerated the expansion of the category of platform workers, who as elsewhere largely remain outside of social protection, and with whom even the definition of 'worker' is often in doubt and contested. The pandemic is likely to increase the tendency towards the application of robots and artificial intelligence, thus leading to further unemployment. The pandemic also had specific gendered impacts as women were disproportionately employed in the service sector and the closure of schools led many female workers to simply withdraw from the labour market.

In conclusion, the contributors to this special issue offer a number of suggestions as to what a post-COVID-19 world might look like and how post-COVID transformations might be channelled in a more progressive direction. Not all the contributors are optimistic about the prospects for such progressive transformations. James and Steger's (2022) comparison of the GFC and COVID-19, for example, is somewhat downbeat due to their observation that the former did not lead to a shift towards positive social transformations and saw minimal reforms to financial markets. James and Steger do, however, note that long-term positive change will depend, as always, on political action. Other contributors to this issue see some potential in the resurgence of state agency and the manner in which support schemes have served to shift the prevailing discourse. Shin (2022) discusses, for example, how in South Korea, the crisis has led to increased calls for alternatives such as the basic income proposal. The latter has been promoted by one of the leading candidates for the 2022 presidential election, Lee Jae-Myung, on the basis of the successful experience of cash payments to citizens in Gyeonggi Province made during the pandemic.

Habibul Haque Khondker (2022) in his commentary highlights the importance of international cooperation. Crucial here is the role of political leaders and their ability to cooperate not just on the pandemic but on the inter-related crises of global warming and social inequality. Stuart et al. (2022) in their analysis of the similar discourses surrounding pandemics and climate change argue that there is a need to tackle false narratives, yet they also emphasize that the broader challenge is the transition towards social conditions that are resilient, healthy, and sustainable. Social and ecological well-being must be prioritized over economic growth. Since the fundamental driver of both climate change and pandemics such as COVID-19 is the economic growth imperative, a post-COVID-19 green recovery would need to move away from an obsession with GDP growth (see the recent Special Issue in *Globalizations* on Economics and Climate Emergency). Above all, it is current power relations that inhibit us from most effectively and justly addressing these crises and thus these power relations must be confronted.

Trommer (2022) argues that post-pandemic recovery requires an ambitious redrawing of global trade relations. In the immediate term, possible reforms of the trade and health nexus within existing institutions include the adoption of the WTO TRIPS waiver and the extension of flexibilities to bilateral and regional trade agreements and to work with non-state actors. This would involve challenging the power relations that uphold the unequal global distribution of products required to fight the pandemic and would include demands for a moratorium on trade negotiations, investment arbitration, and other clauses that directly impact health and social reproductive products and services. Commitments towards health and social reproduction across all instruments of international law should be honoured, including in particular those relating to human rights, labour, and environmental commitments. Broader efforts to shift our thinking about social reproduction, trade, and health require more reflection and consultation among all groups who partake in global trade relations. This includes not only state agents, business representatives, and investors, but also workers, consumers, carers, and citizens.

Recognizing the inter-connected nature of the COVID and climate crisis, Thomas Pogge and Krishen Mehta (2022) put forward a number of concrete proposals inspired by the New Deal reforms for making our social world more resilient. The proposals are not meant to merely tackle the global pandemic but also address the serious vulnerabilities and inequities that it has exposed. The first proposal is a reorganization of the pharmaceutical sector, involving the establishment of a Health Impact Fund that through public funds would reorient the recovery of the costs of innovations away from the sale of branded projects towards public funds. This would motivate pharmaceutical companies to invest in often neglected diseases that impact upon livelihoods in the developing world and shift attention towards fighting communicable diseases at the level of populations. Since the sales price would not be the main source of profit, companies would have strong motivation towards ensuring that their products would reach the poor, thus creating more scope for disease eradication, and there would be less focus on marketing expensive and often inappropriate drugs. The second proposal relates to averting the climate catastrophe through a Green Impact Fund based on similar principles that would promote innovations. Pogge and Mehta also note the need for a shift away from nationally oriented approaches that focus on the extent to which a country is able to reduce emissions domestically towards one that focuses on its external activities, such as the building of coal-powered energy plants overseas. Third, Pogge and Mehta propose the reform of the global tax system in a way that lessens inequality. This involves eliminating fossil fuel subsidies, stemming the abuse of tax havens through a global minimum tax, reducing the risk of recessions through reinstating the Glass–Steagall Act, implementing a financial transaction tax globally, and ensuring fair value for natural resource sales. Pogge and Mehta argue that these reforms are not only transformative and realistic, but that they are also mutually reinforcing, such as with the reform of the global tax system a significant enabler of reforms to the pharmaceutical industry and the addressing of the climate crisis.

In sum, the hopes of countless millions around the globe for progressive future social transformation remain much as they have been for recent years prior to and during the global pandemic (reliant on critical analysis of the present multiple and overlapping crises of capitalist modernity and upon popular mobilization to transform these relations into a more just world). The COVID pandemic did not profoundly alter the existing global system or structure. It revealed again most of the fundamental crisis aspects of the existing global capitalist and international order. There is thus the possibility that, by revealing these fundamentals once again so immediately to vast numbers of people who have suffered as a consequence, that the pandemic will act as a further catalyst for radical social change for years to come.

Notes

1. WHO Coronavirus (COVID-19) Dashboard. Retrieved February 24, 2022, from https://covid19.who.int/.
2. Covid-19 Government Response Tracker. Retrieved February 24, 2022, from https://www.bsg.ox.ac.uk/research/research-projects/covid-19-government-response-tracker.
3. Goldin, I. *COVID-19: How rising inequalities unfolded and why we cannot afford to ignore it*. Retrieved February 24, 2022, from https://theconversation.com/covid-19-how-rising-inequalities-unfolded-and-why-we-cannot-afford-to-ignore-it-161132.
4. Freedom House. *Special Report 2020: Democracy under lockdown*. Retrieved February 24, 2022, from https://freedomhouse.org/report/special-report/2020/democracy-under-lockdown.
5. Nuclear Threat Initiative and Johns Hopkins Center for Health Security. *Global health security index 2019: Building collective action and accountability*. Retrieved February 24, 2022, from https://www.ghsindex.org/wp-content/uploads/2019/10/2019-Global-Health-Security-Index.pdf.
6. Statista. Coronavirus (COVID-19) deaths worldwide per one million population as of February 10, 2022, by country. Retrieved February 24, 2022, from https://www.statista.com/statistics/1104709/coronavirus-deaths-worldwide-per-million-inhabitants/.
7. BBC News. (2021, December 23). *Global Covid vaccine rollout a stain on our soul – Brown*. Retrieved February 24, 2022, from https://www.bbc.co.uk/news/health-59761537.
8. The Economist. (2021, March 27). *As the pandemic rages on, so do protests about it*. Retrieved February 24, 2022, from https://www.economist.com/graphic-detail/2021/03/27/as-the-pandemic-rages-on-so-do-protests-about-it.
9. Nakhaie, R., & Nakhaie, F. S. (2020, 5 July). *Black Lives Matter movement finds new urgency and allies because of COVID-19*. Retrieved February 24, 2022, from https://theconversation.com/black-lives-matter-movement-finds-new-urgency-and-allies-because-of-covid-19-141500.

Disclosure statement

No potential conflict of interest was reported by the author(s).

References

Cooper, L. (2021). *Authoritarian contagion: The global threat to democracy*. Bristol University Press.
Davis, M. (2020). *The monster enters: COVID-19, Avian Flu and the plagues of capitalism*. OR Books.
Denemark, R. A. (2022). Pandemics in global and historical perspective. *Globalizations, 19*(3), 380–396. https://doi.org/10.1080/14747731.2021.1944460
Gerbaudo, P. (2020). The pandemic crowd: Protest in the time of Covid-19. *Journal of International Affairs, 73* (2), 61–75. https://www.jstor.org/stable/26939966

James, P., & Steger, M. B. (2022). On living in an already-unsettled world: COVID as an expression of larger transformation. *Globalizations*, *19*(3), 426–438. https://doi.org/10.1080/14747731.2021.1961460

Jones, L., & Hameiri, S. (2021). COVID-19 and the failure of the neoliberal regulatory state. *Review of International Political Economy*, 1–25. https://doi.org/10.1080/09692290.2021.1892798

Kahl, C. H., & Wright, T. (2021). *Aftershocks: Pandemic politics and the end of the old international order*. St Martin's Press.

Khondeker, H. H. (2022). The post-pandemic world and the prospect for global justic: A commentary. *Globalizations*, *19*(3), 513–517. https://doi.org/10.1080/14747731.2021.1969067

Kumar, R. (2021). Bringing the developmental state back in: Explaining South Korea's successful management of COVID-19. *Third World Quarterly*, *42*(7), 1397–1416. https://doi.org/10.1080/01436597.2021.1903311

Mittelman, J. H. (2022). Global transitioning: Beyond the Covid-19 Pandemic. *Globalizations*, *19*(3), 439–449. https://doi.org/10.1080/14747731.2021.1963201

Nilsen, A. G. (2022). India's pandemic: Spectacle, social murder and authoritarian politics in a lockdown nation. *Gloablizations*, *19*(3), 466–486. https://doi.org/10.1080/14747731.2021.1935019

Pogge, T., & Mehta, K. (2022). A new deal after COVID-19. *Globalizations*, *19*(3), 497–512. https://doi.org/10.1080/14747731.2021.1935020

Sariola, S. (2021). Intellectual property rights need to be subverted to ensure global vaccine access. *BMJ Global Health*, *6*(4), 5–7. https://doi.org/10.1136/bmjgh-2021-005656

Shin, K.-Y. (2022). Work in the post-COVID-19 pandemic: The case of South Korea. *Globalizations*, *19*(3), 487–496. https://doi.org/10.1080/14747731.2021.1969066

Stuart, D., Petersen, B., & Gunderson, R. (2022). Shared pretenses for collective inaction: The economic growth imperative, COVID-19, and climate change. *Globalizations*, *19*(3), 408–425. https://doi.org/10.1080/14747731.2021.1943897

Trommer, S. (2022). Trade, health and social reproduction in a COVID world. *Globalizations*, *19*(3), 397–407. https://doi.org/10.1080/14747731.2021.1964746

van Apeldoorn, B., & de Graaff, N. (2022). The state in global capitalism before and after the Covid-19 crisis. *Contemporary Politics*. Advance online publication. https://doi.org/10.1080/13569775.2021.2022337

Zhou, Y. R. (2022). Vaccine nationalism: Contested relationships between COVID-19 and globalization. *Globalizations*, *19*(3), 450–465. https://doi.org/10.1080/14747731.2021.1963202

Pandemics in global and historical perspective

Robert A. Denemark [ID]

ABSTRACT
Attempts to understand global processes during and after pandemics will benefit from an analysis of historical examples. This work offers a brief review of the impact of various pandemics from about 400 BCE to the present by focusing on (1) states and state strength, (2) class conflict, and (3) global political competition. States are unevenly affected, with capable political units growing in strength and weak units suffering retrenchment. Class conflict increases overall and evidences a multigenerational cycle as labour shortages generate wage pressures. Pandemics alter the global political system given their impact on military conflict, the rise and fall of empires, colonialism, and alterations in power across various regions. A technical note to this work considers challenges in the way we see disease and offers some quick and useful specialized information.

Introduction

Pandemics have been a persistent part of human history, providing evidence of the process of globalization long before it was recognized otherwise. This work identifies 3 areas of human interaction whose developmental paths have been fundamentally affected by pandemics at various points in time: state strength, class conflict, and global political competition. Each provides insights into what we may see during and after our interaction with Covid-19. In a technical note both perceptual challenges relative to disease and useful specialized information are presented. We have faced pandemics before and there are lessons to be learned about relevant social processes.

States and pandemics

The impact of pandemics on states is acute and uneven. In general, a polity with a capable government grows in strength both through the extension of its reach in response to serious challenges, and given the positive impact of successfully managing crisis. Alternatively, polities that are already suffering from decline, have maladaptive leadership, or are corrupt or repressive, will see many of these conditions reinforced. This is especially true in areas like colonies where tenuous legitimacy may be further eroded by pandemics. The role of important actors in commerce or religion may confound state authority.

Success in the face of pandemics is self-reinforcing. The state apparatus grows as a result of the challenge of containing the threat, and if successful, state prerogatives garner further support. This is the story of the fourteenth and fifteenth century city-states that enjoyed their 'golden age' in the

Plague years between 1350 and 1550, as well as nineteenth century governments that dealt with several other diseases (McNeill, 1976, p. 186; McMillen, 2016, p. 5). The city-states of the fourteenth and fifteenth centuries were chartered entities that maintained a range of controls over activities within their boundaries. They were in a unique position to impose restrictions on public interaction that could aid in controlling disease. Three types of activities could prove effective. The first was an enhancement in public sanitation: the treatment of garbage and sewage; the provision of clean water; and the destruction of infected areas (McMillen, 2016, p. 13, 68). Later, as in Britain during the Cholera epidemic of the mid-1800s, Public Health Acts by Parliament and the creation of General Boards of health undertook similar efforts (McMillen, 2016, p. 67). Tuberculosis drove similar efforts in the United States (McMillen, 2016, p. 81).

A second key policy was quarantine. Though contested, the idea that disease was spread by direct contact among people is of great antiquity. It is found in the work of Galen (circa second century CE), who was considered authoritative through the middle-ages, and Procopius, who was court historian to the Byzantine Emperor Justinian I during the outbreak of Bubonic Plague of 541–2 CE. Procopius argued that Plague spread from coastal areas as a result of interaction with traders and worked its way inland (McCormick, 2001, p. 40). Quarantining trading vessels was a key policy in Venice, where ships were ordered to anchor off the port for 40 days (*quaranta giorni* – the genesis of the term quarantine). Similar policies were adopted at select ports and city gates throughout the world.

A third key policy concerned preventive medical action. Inoculation is the most powerful medical tool against infectious diseases. A weakened or partial disease agent is introduced into the body so that it might prepare an immune response for future infections. Though modern vaccination emerged only after the use of microscopes to discover bacteria, the practice existed as early as the eleventh century in China (McNeill, 1976, p. 253). After 1670, with the first look at bacteria through a microscope, to the definitive identification of specific disease agents by Koch in the 1880s, the 'germ theory' took hold and vaccination became both increasingly possible and was often required by the state. Policies on the use of variolation (an early form of inoculation against smallpox), were introduced from Turkey to England in 1721 (McNeill, 1976, pp. 252–253).

Inoculation was not universally popular. State requirements were opposed by several religious creeds in the eighteenth and nineteenth centuries on the grounds that disease was the will of a deity and we should not interfere. States used various methods to reduce opposition. In England, the Royal Family endorsed vaccination against Smallpox (McNeill, 1976, p. 249). George Washington ordered his soldiers vaccinated against Smallpox in 1777, as did Napoleon in 1805 (McNeill, 1976, p. 252). The city of Lexington, Kentucky adopted inoculation against Smallpox in 1803, and it was used in Spain's colonies, including Philippines and Mexico (McNeill, 1976, p. 249). In Japan, importers of vaccines were in the vanguard of opening the country to foreign interaction (McMillen, 2016, p. 39). But the response was often negative. In England vaccination against Smallpox became compulsory after 30,000 deaths in 1836-9, but anti-vaxers rolled back such laws in 1885, 1889, and 1907, as infringements on personal liberties (McMillen, 2016, p. 40).

Where state policies enjoyed success, even if only partial, they earned enhanced legitimacy (Braudel, 1976, p. 333), but efforts were hampered by a range of challenges including 'lax enforcement, porous borders, and the power of merchants to subvert restrictions on their livelihood' (McMillen, 2016, p. 22). Where states broke down, took ineffective actions, or adopted extreme (and unhelpful) policies, the failures were self-reinforcing and led to chaos and decline.

Some polities were simply overwhelmed. Thucydides (c400 BCE/1974: Book 2, 47–55) notes that the plague that struck Athens in about 430 (likely Typhoid) was so destructive that key social norms broke down, bodies were left in the streets, burial rituals disappeared, and individuals engaged in all manner of self-indulgence. Braudel (1981, p. 85) notes a similar fate for municipal governments in some areas of France during the outbreak of Bubonic Plague as officials were among the earliest to flee. (Plague is capitalized when referring to Bubonic Plague and in lower case when used to describe a widespread deadly disease of unknown origin.)

Pandemics led to state failure in several ways. Various authors (Harper, 2017, chapter 3 on Rome; Morris, 2010, p. 301, 396 on China in the second and fourteenth centuries; McNeill, 1976, p. 111, 192 on Central Asia and the Mongols), suggest that as state-controlled trade and tax revenues are reduced, the state could no longer afford to act, and this opens the way for decline or revolution. Ostrogorsky (1966) offers a slightly different model where pandemics facilitate predation by the wealthy that enrages the masses.

Various important groups challenged state-led public health efforts. Though infection tracked trade, commercial interests fought to maintain their prerogatives. Illicit trade was the easiest way to circumvent early efforts at quarantine, and as late as the nineteenth century 'British liberals saw quarantine regulations as an irrational infringement on the principle of free trade, and bent every effort toward the eradication of such traces of tyranny and Roman Catholic folly' (McNeill, 1976, p. 266).

The relationship between commercial interaction, the state, and pandemics, could be complex. Early treatment for the effects of Malaria emerged in the 1650s with the use of the bark of Latin America's Cinchona tree. Exports unfortunately included a great deal of 'counterfeit' bark that was both unhelpful and destroyed confidence in the treatment. The Dutch solved this problem in the 1850s when they began growing Cinchona on colonial plantations in Java (McNeill, 1976, p. 279). Alternatively, in Egypt, which was highly dependent on trade, the Plague killed most of the commercial class. The State stepped in to secure and continue trade relations, but this increased the ruthlessness and corruption of the governing class. Egypt became both more dependent on trade and less capable of benefiting from it (Abu-Lughod, 1989, p. 238).

One of the more pervasive difficulties with state action on pandemics is the role played by religion in public affairs. Religious authorities used scapegoating to deflect uncomfortable questions and weaken old enemies. In Plague-ridden Europe the Flagellants, who beat themselves to atone for unknown sins, called for the killing of Jews as a way to please the deity. They were fighting not only the Plague but the decline in religious belief and the growth of hedonism and mysticism (McNeill, 1976, p. 182). The Catholic Church was in no shape to assist in the actual suppression of diseases, being itself in crisis, so in 1303 the Pope simply declared prayer and killing Jews as acceptable ways to seek divine favour (Morris, 2010, pp. 398–399).

Other religious practices, like pilgrimages and ecclesiastical councils, could also spread disease. This includes Indian pilgrims going to the Cholera-prone lower Ganges; the Catholic Synod in Britain of 664 that spread Bubonic Plague; and annual trips to Mecca that spread Smallpox (Maddicott, 1997; McCormick, 2001, pp. 131–133, 147). Religious ritual could clash directly with the authority of the state:

> In the tiny village of Monte Lupo, in the Tuscan hinterlands, plague arrived in the fall of 1630. Secular and religious official battled over its causes and cures. Religious leaders, along with most of the townspeople, wanted to placate God with a religious procession. Secular health officials, believing that plague was contagious, attempted to restrict such public gatherings and isolate the sick and their families. Riotous violence ensued. (McMillen, 2016, p. 19)

Another major impediment to state policy regarding pandemics was arrogance, often at various points along far-flung empires. In British India the ' ... army and medical corps blindly followed their cultural doctrines' and ignored or rejected input from the local medical community (Cohn, 2012, p. 541). Their actions were not just ineffective but harmful. Eisenberg and Mordechai note

> Although the British made efforts to improve public health in India, a contemporary report noted that 'over fifty years of sanitary work in India' had resulted in 'almost complete failure'. In fact, many of the British infrastructural developments facilitated the spread of disease, so that between 1881 and 1921 life expectancy in India dropped from 25 to 20.1 years. (Eisenberg & Mordechai, 2019, pp. 40–41)

Immediate resentment followed from unprecedented intervention on the bodies of subjects, as well as from the unnecessary burning of personal possessions and homes. Riots broke out in several major cities. In 1897 the British Plague Commissioner was assassinated, colonial authorities had to rescind several rules, and less intrusive (and more effective) methods to control diseases were adopted (McMillen, 2016, p. 28). Cohn (2012, p. 541) notes similar instances in the French African empire. On the island of Tonga the British colonial administration ignored the oncoming Influenza (1918-1919) and blamed local deaths on the moral failings of the natives. Up to 30% of the population of some nearby islands died. The British colonial administration was delegitimized (McMillen, 2016, p. 92). Similar stories emerged in British Africa, where colonial land-use policies drove epidemics of Sleeping Sickness and Malaria, increasing skepticism regarding colonizers and Western medicine (McMillen, 2016, p. 96; McNeill, 1976, p. 48).

Such instances are not unique to the colonial environment. In Russia, Cholera (1830-1) was met by enhanced quarantines and controls on travel that peasants distrusted. As the state destroyed roads and bridges, and forced people into hospitals, peasants attacked state officials, landowners, and hospitals were destroyed (McMillen, 2016, p. 65). In Hungary peasant attacks targeted landowners, priests, doctors, and Jews. The military was mobilized to put down a growing rebellion (Blum, 1978, p. 343).

Even short of violence, the failure of the state can exacerbate a pandemic situation. As the Influenza of 1918 was making its way around the world, San Francisco received advanced warning but failed to mobilize until the disease was present. Hospitals were overwhelmed and the population chaffed under emergency school and entertainment closures, and mask laws. A bomb was sent to the head of the Board of Health. Even the minor reductions in rates of infection and mortality were negated as the population grew tired of the restrictions and began to ignore them. Infection rates rose, exacerbated by the patent medicines that were being pedaled to a naïve populace (Crosby, 2006). Further public efforts at disease control were met with increasing skepticism. All of these processes are visible today.

Class conflict and pandemics

There is a well-understood cyclical process driving class conflict during and in the generations following pandemics. Less well known is the general (secular) increase in class tension that sharpens during pandemic outbreaks: (1) new mechanisms of labour control; (2) alterations in conditions that reduce chances for some pandemic diseases while increasing chances for others; (3) the possible terminal weakening of modes of production; and (4) the intensification of scapegoating along both class and ethnic lines.

The best-known element of pandemic-generated class conflict is the wage cycle. Pandemics have been the single most important driver of population change (Goldstone, 1991, p. 182). As illness takes its toll on the workforce, labour's position is strengthened. During the Antonine Plague of 160, for example, Egyptian wages rose significantly (Morris, 2014). Historically, such demands have generated a political response. When the Plague of 541–2 led to increasing labour costs, especially among sailors, the emperor Justinian froze wages (McCormick, 2001, p. 109). Edicts were promulgated in Constantinople during a plague outbreak in 543 condemning wage and price increases (Cohn, 2012, p. 22). In response to Plague-based wage increases in England we find the 'Ordinance of Labourers' (1349) and the 'Statute of Labourers' (1351) that together capped and then decreased pay and made it illegal in some instances to decline employment regardless of the wage offered (McMillen, 2016, p. 14). Similar wage control efforts are noted in Italy, where laws to restrict rural labour mobility were enacted (1348 and 1387), and curbs were place on landowners who were offering extra incentives (like free meals) (Jones, 1966, p. 362, 426-7). In Scandinavia, laws emerged to compel the homeless to work on farms and these remained in place long after the pandemic eased (Bolin, 1966).

Postan (1966, p. 609) suggested that efforts at wage controls were only partly successful. But as pandemics recede and populations rise, labour is no longer scarce, and the position of workers and sharecroppers deteriorates. The result is a cycle of class conflict that finds labour on the ascent after pandemics, and on the decline as populations are re-established.

Along with the tension of the wage cycle, there are four more secular impacts of pandemics on class conflict. First, a shortage of labour is not immediately made up for by population growth. As wages rise we see alternative methods of controlling labour. Debt peonage is adopted as a strategy (McNeill, 1976, p. 206), and slavery emerges (McCormick, 2001, p. 512). Second, a change in labour conditions, together with a climate alteration toward cooling temperatures after the Bubonic Plague in fourteenth century Europe, altered behaviours in ways that impact subsequent communicable diseases. The relationships between humans and pathogens are complex and here we see the impact of both pandemics on class struggle and of changing labour conditions on the rise of pandemic diseases. Rising wages along with cooling temperatures led workers to the purchase more woollen goods. This reduced the prevalence of epidemic Yaws (spread by skin contact) but increased the prevalence of Typhus (spread by fleas) (McNeill, 1976, p. 179). Pandemics may have different impacts on other pandemic diseases, only some of which effect class relations. Epidemic leprosy in Europe was reduced by Bubonic Plague-induced deaths of entire leper colonies. AIDS weakens immune responses and allowed for the return of pandemic tuberculosis (TB). TB was the leading cause of death in Europe in the nineteenth century, but because of AIDS it now kills more people (mostly in the global south) than ever before (McMillen, 2016, p. 86).

Third, we note a debate regarding the impact of pandemic-induced labour shortages on the decline of feudalism. While feudal labour services were already in retreat, the demographic effects of the Plague accelerated this process significantly. This was explicit in Spain (Smith, 1966, p. 437) and noted more generally throughout Europe (Genicot, 1966, p. 713, 731). Postan reviews a series of post-Plague peasant revolts (circa 1381) and suggests the 'final breakup of medieval serfdom' (1966, p. 608). The role of the Plague in ending feudalism is also noted by Morris (2014). Campbell avoids the debate over feudalism per se, but concludes that in the early 1340s, as Plague 'erupted with explosive force' the result was that 'Europe's already floundering socio-economic regime was terminally undermined and a long downturn initiated upon whose course war, climate change and disease continued to exercise a powerful influence' (Campbell, 2016, pp. 328–329). Little could be more relevant to class conflict than the decline of an entire mode of production.

Fourth, a general (non-cyclical) sharpening of class conflict emerged across several pandemics given the desire of people to affix blame for their misfortunes. Upheaval followed the cessation of the bread rations distributed to Rome's poor in 618 due to the destruction of both the capacity to import grain from the periphery, and the ability of the state to collect sufficient revenues to pay for it (McCormick, 2001, p. 783). Braudel notes the suspicion generated by the rich when they fled stricken cities and notes the 'social massacres of the poor' that result (1976, pp. 333–334). He quotes Sartre's suggestion that 'The plague only exaggerates the relationship between the classes: it strikes at the poor and spares the rich' (Braudel, 1979/1981 vol 3, p. 85). In France, Cholera was viewed as a plot designed by the wealthy to get rid of the poor (McMillen, 2016, p. 64). Even rumours of Plague could sharpen class struggle (McNeill, 1976, p. 172).

In Byzantium, famine and plague followed the bad winter of 927-8. The wealthy started buying up peasant land at discounted prices. Social unrest increased and the emperor denounced the practice and instituted laws to prohibit it, but this only slowed the process. By 967 a new pro-landowner emperor was on the throne, and the social upheaval that landlessness created contributed to the eventual collapse of the Byzantine empire (Ostrogorsky, 1966, pp. 217–221)

Class conflict is also heightened by the fact that post-plague income distribution is highly uneven. In the post-Bubonic Plague 1400s wealth was concentrated among survivors, albeit unequally and, for labour, precariously (McCormick, 2001, p. 753). Lopez (1967, p. 395) notes the bifurcation of quality production following the Plague. There were luxury goods, and the cheapest possible goods, and little in between.

Scapegoating is a recurrent theme of communities under threat and is often used deflect class conflict. Pandemic's scapegoats have included Jews, immigrants, and homosexuals who were targeted during periods of Plague, Cholera, and AIDS respectively. McMillen (2016, p. 12) estimates that around 1000 Jewish communities were destroyed by their neighbours during the Plague years.

Immigrants constitute another group that is often set upon in difficult times. Recognition of a link between rural-to-urban immigration and disease emerges as early as 400 BCE (Thucydides, c400 BCE/1974, Book 2, 51–53). Diseases like Cholera, caused by unclean water, helped mark immigrants not as victims but as carriers (McMillen, 2016, p. 66). The same is often true of Dysentery and Smallpox (Russell, 1969, p. 54). Tuberculosis is another disease blamed on immigrants because of its ability to spread more quickly in cramped living conditions among individuals who lack sufficient food. TB was Europe's deadliest disease in the nineteenth and early twentieth centuries, killing far more individuals than the Plague, and rates were far higher among minority populations (McMillen, 2016, p. 78).

Migration may spread disease in other ways, creating or exacerbating already fraught class relations. During the colonial period, Africans from inland areas were forced to work near coasts. They were infected with Malaria by mosquitoes, which they brought home at the end of their work detail and spread to others via local mosquito populations (McMillen, 2016, p. 51). Areas already infected saw disease rates increase. Those without Malaria suffered its introduction. A similar tale, if at the global level, might be told of AIDS, which is thought to have made the transition from an animal host to a human host in Central Africa in the 1920s as a result of a hunter allowing animal blood to penetrate a wound. In Africa, AIDS is spread primarily by heterosexual relations, but in the West it was a disease that spread mostly through needle-sharing, transfusions, and homosexual relations. AIDS was therefore identified as a disease of the drug-addicted, the sick, or those of 'alternative' lifestyles. Funding and treatment lagged as a result, as did attention to the heterosexual modes of transmission more relevant to control efforts in Africa (McMillen, 2016, pp. 103–109).

Post-pandemic class conflict is indelibly marked with the relations that emerged during the period of rampant illness. The wage cycle may take a generation or two to rebound in favour of owners. Technology developed to help cope with labour shortages does not disappear, and this may lead to quicker wage suppression (Crosby, 2006, p. 283). Scapegoating may abate but it is a persistent strategy that strengthens with use. Lingering hatreds – of 'foreigners' or 'migrants' or 'the wealthy' – will be quicker to emerge in subsequent instances. Communities that were destroyed, individuals who were killed, and institutions that were delegitimized, are not resurrected. Lands that were abandoned may be repopulated, though after the Plague of the fourteenth century it took upwards of 100–150 years before agriculture fully recovered. Pandemics exacerbate class conflict in both the immediate period and in multigenerational timeframes.

Pandemics and global political change

Pandemics manifest themselves at the global political level as well. Specific battles and wars may be determined by the health of troops. The fall of established empires and the rise of new colonial expansion are implicated, and alterations in the power of various regions in the global system may be at stake.

Pandemics often begin with armies camped in far-off locations, as was the case for the Romans in Mesopotamia, the Chinese in Myanmar, and the Mongols across Eurasian grasslands. The Influenza Pandemic of 1918 was labelled the 'Spanish Flu' because Spain was neutral in the ongoing world war and its press was allowed to report on it. In reality, the 'Spanish' Flu is often argued to have begun at a military base in rural Kansas and war-time conditions helped it spread and led to restrictions on information about it. Far earlier instances include the (unknown) disease suffered by the Greeks besieging Troy (Crosby, 2006, p. 283). In 161–2 nearly one third of Chinese troops died when a pestilence broke out among them on the northwest frontier (Morris, 2010, p. 296). Spanish troops contracted Typhus in Cyprus in 1490 (McNeill, 1976, p. 220). In all these cases the diseases reduced military capacity and spread back to the metropole. Pandemics are often suggested to emerge from war and trade, but as Morris (2010, p. 347) notes, the two go together. Traders regularly visit military encampments to supply food and other necessities, and spread diseases as a result.

Pandemics have made the difference between military victory and defeat. Athens was badly weakened by pandemic illness during the Peloponnesian War, and the history of Greece, and perhaps the entire region would have been quite different if the results had been otherwise (McNeill, 1976, p. 105). Abu-Lughod notes that the Plague weakened Genoa and Venice in the midst of their commercial competition, and each militarized immediately thereafter to fight over the post-Plague spoils (1989, p. 127). In 1526 the French Army had to withdraw from the siege of Naples, and other sieges were abandoned during the War of the Spanish Succession because of illness. In 1802–3 the French faced Yellow Fever during the Haitian Revolution that accounted for the loss of 80% of their troops (Smallman-Raynor & Cliff, 2004, p. 118). In the 1820s and 1830s the Russian army spread Cholera to Persia, Turkey, Poland, then it travelled through the Baltic to England, Canada, the US, and reached Mexico by 1833 (McNeill, 1976, p. 263). Dysentery inflicted 10 times more casualties on the British military than did their enemies in Crimea, and five times the casualties as their opponents in the Boer War (McNeill, 1976, p. 284). The Nazis used Typhus to do much of their dirty-work in the extermination camps that housed Jews, Roma, Gays, the infirm, and all manner of dissenters. Research on Typhus was conducted in such camps because of a ready supply of disposable test subjects. The Nazi habit of promoting individuals based on fidelity to the party and not technical competence allowed subordinate staff in one major laboratory to sabotage their own (successful) vaccine heading to Nazi troops on their already precarious Eastern Front (Allen, 2014).

Empires were at stake as well. In the second century both the Roman (Morris, 2010, p. 302, 317), and the Han (Lopez, 1967, p. 29) empires suffered greatly. Gibbon (1776/1994, p. 731) notes that

Justinian's attempts to enlarge, or at least codify the Eastern Roman Empire were defeated by the sixth century Plague. The same Plague helped weaken the social fabric of the Byzantine Empire (McMillen, 2016, p. 8). (A sophisticated counterargument by Eisenberg and Mordechai (2019) raises questions about this 'maximalist view' and its tendencies toward 'catastrophism'.) More recent disease outbreaks are better understood and their impacts on empires are more easily traced. As an example, epidemic diseases took the lives of so many French soldiers in the Caribbean that Napoleon decide to sell Louisiana instead of pursuing plans for greater empire in North America (McNeill, 1976, p. 266). Plagues of various sorts led to declines in population, commerce, and tax revenue, leaving Empires weakened and vulnerable.

Pandemic disease was also a potent and often self-consciously utilized weapon of empire. In places like Australia and New Zealand the colonists simply had to arrive to spread the Influenza that would decimate the indigenous population (McMillen, 2016, p. 91). McNeill repeats the charge that Native North Americans were gifted blankets infected with Smallpox to wipe them out (McNeill, 1976, p. 251). Chase-Dunn et al. (2007, pp. 132–133) follow Mike Davis in noting how occasional drought spread famine and epidemics. These were capitalized upon by imperial powers seeking to integrate peripheral areas more closely into markets or impose formal colonial status. The result was unprecedented levels of death in Brazil, India, China, and the Philippines.

Nothing, however, compares to the carnage that resulted from the intrusion of Europeans into Latin America. Some 60–90 percent of the indigenous population died over a 50-year period (Livi-Bacci, 2008: Chapter 3). The despondence that followed made it easy for imperialists to change the social and religious beliefs of those who survived (McNeill, 1976, p. 204). Bentley (2006, p. 404) concludes that ' … these massive transoceanic epidemics may have caused more deaths than any other agent in human history.'

Pandemics also play a role in the relative dominance of different core regions. Cities declined relative to hinterlands (Abu-Lughod, 1989, p. 95). The pandemic that returned to Rome from Mesopotamia ' … inaugurated a process of continued decay of the population of Mediterranean lands that lasted, despite local recoveries, for more than half a millennium' (McNeill, 1976, p. 116). Russell adds that Malaria must be held partly responsible for the decline of the Mediterranean countries in both medieval and early modern times (Russell, 1969, p. 53). As the Mediterranean declined, dominance shifted to the North of Europe (McNeill, 1976, p. 131). Nomadic groups rose in Arabia with the decline of settled states (McMillen, 2016, p. 9). McMillen (2016, p. 83) also notes that Plague hobbled western Mediterranean shipping and left mostly those ships from the Eastern Mediterranean to trade and raid. The Champagne Trade Fairs of northeastern France, once a vital trade node and source of considerable local wealth, were effectively shut down when Plague weakened Genoa and Venice – whose traders had provided the eastern goods that made the Fairs so valuable (Abu-Lughod, 1989, p. 73). New sources of raw materials and new shortages helped some areas to rise and others to fall irrespective of actions that were being taken locally (Abu-Lughod, 1989, p. 96).

An excellent example of the sort of regional changes that could be wrought is offered by McMillen in a discussion of native North Americans:

> Smallpox rearranged the ethnic landscape of native North America. … Devastated by smallpox in the 1630s, the Iroquois increased their "mourning wars" – the capture of enemies to replace Iroquois dead – against their longtime foe, the Huron. Smallpox ravaged the Iroquois; it nearly decimated the Huron. And this, combined with Iroquois military prowess, allowed the Iroquois to emerge as the dominant power. The same epidemic forced the Sauk and Fox to seek refuge further west among other groups, fostering the creation of new ethnic identities. Smallpox kept coming and coming, rearranging the

ethnic order again and again. Differential mortality left some groups weak and other strong The Ani-sinaabe-speaking Monsoni, powerful middlemen in the beaver trade by the 1670s, were nearly wiped out by smallpox in the 1730s; survivors drifted to other groups, and by the end of the century they ceased to be a discrete people. Into the void stepped people like the northern Ojibwa. (McMillen, 2016, pp. 35–36)

Conclusion

Crosby (2006, p. 281) concludes: 'Humanity was not genetically prepared for the environment that it started creating ten or so thousand years ago. It is a major irony that humans are not well adapted to the environment they have created.' Pandemics play a role in three key socio-political processes: state strength, class conflict, and global political change. In each case we see important implications, and this conclusion only provides a short sketch of the many permutations and examples that can be offered.

In the area of state strength we see the sharpening of the stakes in the process of maintaining sufficient latitude to intervene in society, but only if in an effective way. Effective intervention strengths the state. Ineffective intervention leads to further weakening of both society and the state. Policies like quarantine, inoculation, sanitation, and the ability to control special interests like commercial classes and religious leaders, have been applied historically and can lead to success. If the state cannot or will not engage in such activities, previously powerful leaders can fall, as we saw in the elections in the US in 2020, and state institutions can be delegitimized.

Class conflict is expected to increase during pandemics for both cyclical and secular reasons. Wage cycles, exacerbated by the development of new modes of labour control and of labour-saving technology, promise long-term instability. The gap between rich and poor, and the politization of the differences, increases class friction. It may be difficult to see the Covid-19 pandemic as critical to wage structures given the ability of state controls and medical science to mitigate death rates. None-theless shortages in education, the service economy, and health care have already been noted (Jacobs, 2020; Politi & Fedor, 2020; Rogers, 2021), and the negative effects of the pandemic on edu-cation are 'even more marked for children from marginalized communities or disadvantaged groups' (Jack & Staton, 2021, p. 4).

Perhaps the most sweeping treatment of pandemics and class analysis is offered by Karatasli (2020) who suggests

> Government responses to the Covid-19 pandemic reveal once again that when rulers around the world realize that they need to make a choice between risking either capital accumulation or human lives, most opt for risking/sacrificing the latter without much hesitation.

Aside from the costs of partial closure and public health efforts, Karatasli notes the advantages to capital in advanced countries of pushing pandemic deaths into the 'shadows' of the private (as opposed to the public) realm, and the relatively low costs to 'the economy' of deaths of older citi-zens who consume less and collect expensive pensions. In support of his analysis he notes that states of the semi-periphery that depend on industrial production have often taken more effective action than far wealthier, post-industrial core areas.

Finally, scapegoating emerged in both its class and especially its ethnic modes, first marking those of Asian ancestry for poor treatment given COVID-19's origins in Wuhan, but reflecting also on immigrant labour. Generating such hatreds can take the place of instituting necessary health policies.

Global political change is also sharpened. Obvious propaganda designed to 'blame' one country or another for a pandemic tend to backfire and are not particularly successful in avoiding the ire of populations whose leadership fail to take appropriate and effective action at home. Military preparedness suffers more in those states with both a larger and more dispersed security apparatus, and the need to depend upon it. Political squabbles, the desire to shorten supply chains, and assure critical resources, generate realignments of various sorts. Hungary broke ranks with the rest of Europe and purchased vaccines from China and Russia, driving an even deeper wedge into the EU. Mahbubani (2020) and Schake (2020) argue that the pandemic's impact on US politics served to undermine US leadership and render globalization more China-centric. Gabuev (2020) outlines the many ways in which the current pandemic is pushing China and Russia together to oppose various US efforts, and simultaneously strengthening the need for states in Asia to follow China. And not surprisingly, economic growth in the global south was hit harder, and will recover more slowly, than in the global north.

The interaction of pandemic disease with other social and natural processes, especially climate change, raises a variety of concerns for the near future as well. Of the authors noted in this work, the vast majority link pandemics to climate. Temperature changes effect clothing styles, building materials, sleeping conditions, cleaning conventions, the mating habits of various herd animals, rodents, birds, and disease organisms, along with population movements and agricultural productivity and practices. Generally cooling temperatures and altered rainfall patterns (not seasonal changes) are implicated in the spread of Bubonic Plague, Malaria, and the full range of diseases that are passed from animals to humans either by proximity or in the food chain. Generally rising temperatures are hypothesized to have an even larger impact mostly because of the changing geographic ranges of insects and disease-carrying animals.

The historical implications of pandemic disease for states, classes, and global actors offers significant insight into our current situation, and what is likely to follow.

Technical note

Pandemics: a users guide

Scholars tend to ignore or discount disease as pertinent to social developments. Students of pandemics suggest that this may be the result of aversion to disease, or our strong preference for explanations that focus on human agency (McMillen, 2016; McNeill, 1976). We could add the fact that the definitions are contentious, the death tolls are horrific, and the biology of human pathogens is unfamiliar and complex. Serious diseases of the sort that become pandemics are episodic, but not rare. They ought to be considered part of the human condition. We must deal with misperceptions about disease, along with some technical information, in order to recognize and understand their historical, contemporary, and likely future implications.

Misperceptions

Virulent diseases emerge from several sources and have complex relationships with a variety of life forms. It is easier to understand them if we (1) avoid thinking of humans as unitary organisms that are (2) intentionally infected by other life forms, and that (3) this takes place in an environment characterized by stable predator-and-prey dynamics.

Contrary to our common-knowledge understandings, humans are not unitary life forms. Our physical existence is intertwined with those of others biological agents that we adopt and have come to depend upon over the long evolutionary term. For every uniquely 'human' cell in our bodies there are 10 'other' cells cohabitating with us that facilitate core human processes like nutrition, energy transformation, and even protection against infectious diseases (Blaser, 2006). We have defenses from invasion by other life forms, but the protection is not perfect even when oriented toward entities our bodies identify as dangerous. We take 'foreign' entities on board when we interact with different people, experience new climates, deal with new animals, devise new agricultural practices, or extend the range or density of our settlements.

Second, not all pathogens should be thought of as other forms of life. Most bacteria can exist independently of humans, often in the soil or other animals, and may be considered a life form. But viruses have no metabolism, nor can they reproduce outside a living host. On their own they are non-viable and are not considered a 'life form'.

Neither viruses nor other disease organisms act with intent. Diseases are not generally 'looking for' human hosts to provide them with a viable future. Humans may not be their natural habitat at all. In many cases, we are little more than collateral damage. Pathogens may prove too virulent and destroy all human hosts. Likewise, they may be too weak and fail to propagate. Some are much better suited to parasitizing non-human life forms such that human infection is accidental or opportunistic. In optimal cases, it can still take humans a century or two to generate even a tenuous equilibrium between the virulence of a pathogen and the resilience of humans both initially and over time.

Third, both humans and pathogenic agents evolve – that is – they alter randomly and those mutations that afford them an advantage allow for superior reproductive rates, while those that do not aid the individual will fail to survive. As both pathogen and host may mutate, the complexity of the situation increases exponentially (Chase-Dunn et al., 2010; Devezas, 2020).

To further complicate things, the environment within which this mutually evolving interaction takes place also changes or evolves. Most obvious is the tendency toward alterations in base temperatures. Figure 1 comes from the work of Chase-Dunn et al. (2010) and attempts to provide a sense of the complexity and interaction of various networks that are usually considered separately.

It may be possible to begin an analysis with the population variable (upper right), about which we have a vast literature, and attempt to validate its relationships with the other elements that are identified above. Of particular interest might be data on inequality as an indicator of several human sociocultural elements identified in Figure 1, and which has been the focus of recent scholarship that pursues elements of its growth, reduction, social interactions, and measurement back into pre-history (Kohler & Smith, 2018; Scheidel, 2017). Other empirical efforts at social analysis over the long historical term have proven both possible and popular (eg. Morris, 2013, 2014). Biology allows us to peer into even farther back into such phenomena (Eisenberg & Mordechai, 2019; Pearce-Duvet, 2006).

It would be especially useful to address questions of causation. In what ways do social changes facilitate pandemics, and vice versa. Scheidel (2017, pp. 10–11) purposely avoids discussions of the ways inequality might foster the violence, state failure, and pandemics that tend to level the social order perhaps to avoid being mired in complexity. Others could begin to untangle those processes. Further work might build on existing literature to establish other critical relationships as regards war, resource depletion, or urbanization in relation to microbial change and human genetic alterations such as immune responses. Hypothetically we might be able to tie state strength, class conflict, and global political change (socio-political variables identified in this work) together in a systematic

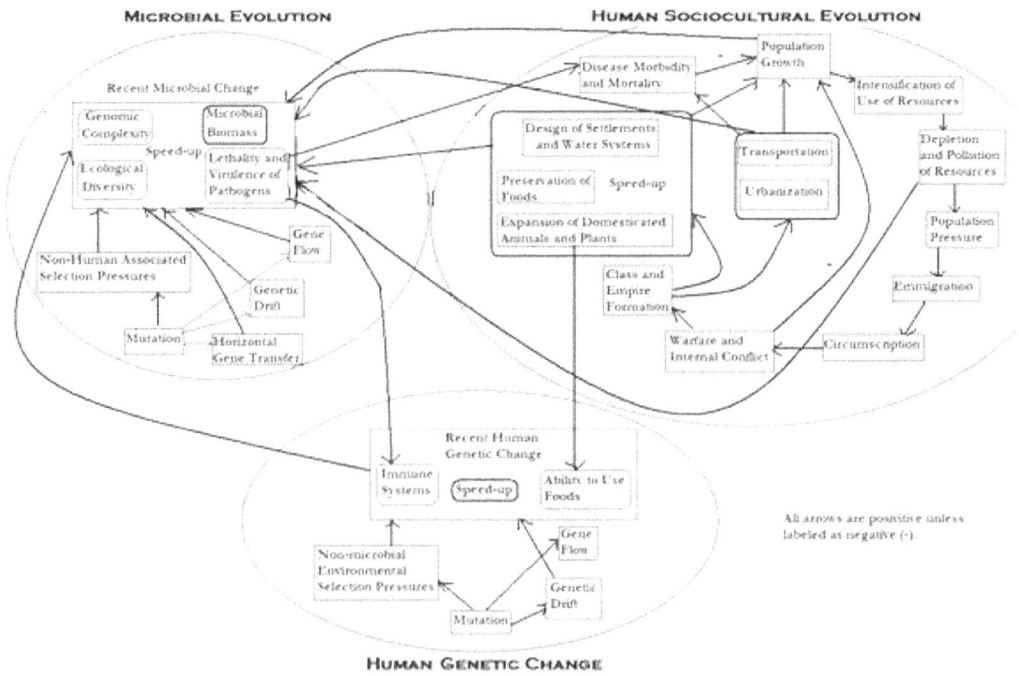

Figure 1. Conceptual diagram of causes within and between three realms.

manner. But the contingent nature of the variables, the lack of certain important data, and the inherent complexity created by so many possible linkages and feedbacks, might make validation efforts at the level of the broader model impossible at this time.

Definitions

Pandemics can be challenging to define. An epidemic is a disease that is confined to one region. A pandemic occurs over a wide geographical area and affects a significant proportion of the world's population. Pandemics emerge from epidemics. Of course a disease that sweeps through China or Russia might be called an epidemic as it appears in only one country, while the same disease covering the same space in western Europe would traverse a dozen borders and probably be considered a pandemic. A similarly expansive disease in the Global South might simply be ignored. An excellent way to avoid these problems is to consider a definition that is more disease-centric. Following McMillen (2016, p. 1), pandemics might be defined as diseases that bring severe symptoms, encounter minimal immunity in the population, have high rates of infectiousness and contagiousness – all with a wide geographic extension (McMillen, 2016, p. 1). This definition is hardly well-focused, but provides a less arbitrary basis than those driven by a concern with political boundaries.

Causes and treatments of pandemic disease

Disease is caused when pathogens enter a body, attach to host cells, and produce destructive toxins or enzymes. Human diseases emerge from 5 types of pathogens, but only 3 have been implicated in pandemics. The two most important are single celled organisms (bacteria or protozoans), and nucleic acids (viruses or retroviruses). Multi-celled worms or flukes are the source of another pandemic disease: Schistosomiasis. Fungi and prions are also sources of human disease but have not generated pandemics.

Bacteria and protozoans are single-celled organisms that may live in the soil or animals, including humans. They are identified (and named) by their shapes (bacillus are rod-shaped, coccus are spherical, and spirillum are helical). Unlike human cells, bacterial cells lack a membrane-delimited nucleus. They may be attacked with chemicals (anti-biotics) that target the synthesis of their cell walls, proteins, or other of their elements. Because human cells are structured differently, certain compounds may attack bacterial or protozoan cells uniquely. Once a bacteria or protozoa is linked to a specific disease, anti-biotics may be identified and used without undue harm to the patient. Bacterial pandemics include Tuberculosis, Bubonic Plague, Malaria, Typhoid fever, Leprosy, and Typhus.

Viruses and retroviruses are strands of DNA or RNA surrounded by a protein coat, and they sometimes acquire a covering of material from the host cell as well. Viruses inject themselves into specific host cells and get that cell to reproduce their DNA or viral proteins. These are released to infect more cells, sometimes killing the host cell in the process. Retroviruses use a specific enzyme to copy the RNA genome into DNA that takes over the host cell. Retroviruses can hide for long periods of time, and like all RNA viruses, tend to mutate frequently, which confounds attempts to eradicate them. Since viruses hide in, sometimes cover themselves with, and reproduce within human cells, the substances that would kill them are also toxic to their human hosts. There are some antiviral drugs that target virus-specific enzymes, often to inhibit replication. This is an ongoing area of research. Viral pandemics include Influenza, Smallpox, HIV/AIDS, and variations on SARS including Covid-19.

Flukes are small worms that enter a body and grow, using human tissues to support themselves. Though not well represented among pandemics, worm-based Schistosomiasis has been important historically, especially in areas where agricultural production in standing water takes place. Schistosomiasis currently infects about 230 million people on multiple continents (Pennisi, 2018). It may be controlled with medications that kill the worms.

The definitive medical intervention against communicable disease is vaccination. The body has a natural system of protecting itself that is initiated when a damaging foreign entity (an antigen) gains entry. Special cells (macrophages) are designed to destroy the foreign entity and display bits of it (like its unique proteins) on their outer cell walls. Other cells (T-cells and B-cells) use these bits to identify and generate an attack against similar intruders elsewhere in the body – releasing lymphokines that stimulate even more cells to participate in the response. T-cells attach to infected cells and destroy them. Other cells produce toxins that target the pathogen itself. B-cells produce proteins that recognize and bind to the pathogen, marking it for attack. Other B-cells become 'memory B-cells' that respond to a specific antigen by generating a quick response in case of reinfection. The quick response is often sufficient to ward off a disease, which is why vaccination is effective. The process is far more difficult if the pathogen gains a foothold, hides in human cells, or mutates rapidly, which is why vaccines for viruses and retroviruses are so difficult to create.

The lethality of pandemic diseases

Pandemic diseases have generated astonishing death tolls. We cannot provide a definitive list of deadly pandemics without so many caveats regarding data collection that eyes would glaze over.

Further, raw figures are unhelpful given changing global and regional population figures. Just as an example, we know the Bubonic Plague of the fourteenth century is estimated to have taken at least two hundred million lives, suggesting a death rate throughout western Europe of approximately 30–40 percent. One hundred and seventy years later Smallpox claimed some 56 million lives, eventually killing some 60–90 percent of the population of America. In 1775 another Smallpox outbreak in North America infected 95% of the population and one in seven died. Lesser-known pandemics have also generated high death tolls. Five percent of the Hungarian population died of Cholera in 1831. The Influenza of 1918–9 took 40–50 million lives. These figures are hardly definitive, and unfortunately western-biased. When looking for general figures one might begin at websites like https://www.livescience.com/worst-epidemics-and-pandemics-in-history.html titled '20 of the worst epidemics and pandemics in history' that organizes information on pandemics by instance (e.g. 'The Plague of Justinian'), or https://en.wikipedia.org/wiki/Pandemic titled 'Notable Outbreaks' that organizes information based on disease. The figures are astounding.

The genesis of pandemic diseases

Many diseases that infect humans come from animals. The process of transference is called zoonosis, and is often noted in the wake of the human domestication of various animals starting some 14,000 years ago. Animal pathogens are often capable of finding new hosts, or mutating in a way that allows them to do so. The closer the proximity (i.e. in settled agriculture as opposed to nomadic herding), the easier the transfer. The more types of animals that join the community (and a typical farm might include various chickens, pigs, horses, cattle, sheep, and goats, along with masses of vermin, while early towns and cities might not have been all that different), the more types of diseases might be transferred. Agricultural pursuits in new areas (as in virgin grasslands where rodent colonies might be disturbed), or in standing water (as with rice cultivation), increase the likelihood of the transference of disease organisms. Examples include Influenza from birds and swine; HIV/AIDS from chimpanzees, and Smallpox from Camelpox or Cowpox (whose name notwithstanding is actually a rodent disease) (Pearce-Duvet, 2006).

The relationship between agriculture and infectious diseases is complex. Pearce-Duvet (2006) uses genetic evidence to question the traditional idea that domesticated animals pass diseases directly to humans. Instead she notes that agriculture and domesticated animal herds may increase disease by

> (a) changing the transmission ecology of pre-existing human pathogens; (b) increasing the success of pre-existing pathogen vectors, resulting in novel interactions between humans and wildlife; (c) providing a stable conduit for human infestation by wildlife diseases by means of domesticated animals (p. 378)

Influenza is an excellent example. Influenza from wild birds affects pigs and poultry, which host human viruses as well. The resulting admixture allows for various forms of viral mutation and cross-contamination (Pearce-Duvet, 2006, p. 379). (Note, however, that the 1918 Influenza transferred to humans directly from wild birds.)

Disease may also be passed from animals to humans by 'vectors' defined as organisms that transfer pathogens from one host to another. Plague was passed from fleas to rats and other rodents, and when the rats came into close contact with humans the fleas would pass along the pathogen. Rodent colonies are endemic homes to Plague. Plague could also be passed via droplets from the breadth. Another example is Malaria, which is passed along by mosquitoes who pick up the disease in the form of the protozoon *Plasmodium* and pass it to subsequent victims. The key to control of the disease, as in many other cases, is environmental (Burney, 1995). As humans work to alter the landscape (building irrigation systems or forcing labour into areas of active infection) they provide additional homes for mosquitoes. Clearing standing water where mosquitos breed is crucial to control. Enhanced global connectivity through all manner of travel is implicated as well (Devezas, 2020, p. 2). Burney concludes that that the biggest impact of humans on the earth was the movement of living things that 'destabilize local abiotic environments' (1995, p. 261).

Diseases may also be waterborne or foodborne. Among waterborne diseases we note Schistosomiasis, which McNeill suggests was so widespread and so debilitating as to cripple populations and leave them open to individual or collective predation (1976, p. 45). Moving into new areas, or seeking new food sources, enhances the transfer of disease to humans as well. The eating of civets (a species related to mongooses) in southern China transferred SARS from bats to humans (Roos, 2004). Covid-19 likely transferred from bats as well.

As important as it is to understand some of the science that underlies pandemics, they remain social phenomena. War, poverty, inequality, official disregard, forced migration, trade, travel, counterfeiting medications, avarice, responses to climate change, agricultural expansion, the use of disease agents to decimate opposition populations, the search for 'unique' foods, and the flow of refugees are all implicated in new or resurgent diseases that may grow into pandemics. McMillen (2016, p. 2) notes that tuberculosis was once Europe's leading cause of death. Public health efforts and medications have made it rare in that Global North. Yet it remains, for all our knowledge, a major cause of death in the Global South. Medication and information are not enough. The social challenges that help give rise to pandemics both pre-date outbreaks and are likely to carry over, or become more acute, in the post-pandemic world.

Acknowledgements

I am grateful to Thomas Hall, Joseph Wald z"l, and David Wilkinson for many years of fascinating discussions on a variety of related subjects. Christopher Chase-Dunn was kind enough to give permission to use Figure 1. In the 38 years I've been submitting articles for peer review I have never enjoyed three more stimulating, challenging, or helpful responses from reviewers. Though I could not follow up all their suggestions, this work is far better for their input. I am especially grateful to those members of my family involved in science and medicine for their patient tutelage: Cynthia Denemark, Eric Denemark, Howard Denemark z"l, Grace Tannin Denemark z"l, and Jonathan Mizrahi.

Disclosure statement

No potential conflict of interest was reported by the author(s).

ORCID

Robert A. Denemark ⓘ http://orcid.org/0000-0001-5764-8885

References

Abu-Lughod, J. (1989). *Before European hegemony*. Oxford University Press.

Allen, A. (2014). *The fantastic laboratory of Dr. Weigl*. W.W. Norton.

Bentley, J. (2006). The New World history. In L. Kramer, & S. Maza (Eds.), *A companion to Western historical thought* (pp. 393–416). Blackwell.

Blaser, M. (2006). Who are we? *EMBO Reports*, 7(10), 956–960. https://doi.org/10.1038/sj.embor.7400812

Blum, J. (1978). *The end of the old order in rural Europe*. Princeton University Press.

Bolin, S. (1966). Scandinavia. In M. M. Postan (Ed.) *The Cambridge economic history of Europe* (Vol. 1. 2nd ed., pp. 633–659). Cambridge University Press.

Braudel, F. (1976). *The Mediterranean and the Mediterranean World in the age of Philip II* (Vol. 2, Sian Reynolds, Trans.). Harper Colophon. (Original work published 1949)

Braudel, F. (1981). *Civilization and capitalism 15th-18th century* (Vols 3, Sian Reynolds, Trans.). Harper and Row. (Original work published 1979)

Burney, D. (1995). Historical perspectives on human-assisted biological invasions. *Evolutionary Anthropology: Issues, News, and Reviews*, 4(6), 216–221. https://doi.org/10.1002/evan.1360040605

Campbell, B. (2016). *The great transition: Climate, disease and society in the late-medieval world*. Cambridge University Press.

Chase-Dunn, C., Hall, T., & Turchin, P. (2007). World-systems in the biogeosphere: Urbanization, state formation, and climate change since the Iron Age. In A. Hornborg, & C. Crumley (Eds.), *The world system and the earth system* (pp. 132–148). Left Coast Press.

Chase-Dunn, C., Sachs, J., Turchin, P., & Hanneman, R. (2010). Spiraling coupled human and biotic systems: microbial and sociocultural coevolution since the Bronze Age. Institute for Research on World-Systems paper #95. Retrieved November 1, 2020, from https://irows.ucr.edu/papers/irows95/irows95.htm

Cohn, S. (2012). Pandemics: Waves of disease, waves of hate from the Plague of Athens to A.I.D.S. *Historical Research*, 85(230), 535–555. https://doi.org/10.1111/j.1468-2281.2012.00603.x

Crosby, A. (2006). Infectious diseases as ecological and historical phenomena, with special reference to the Influenza Pandemic of 1918-1919. In A. Hornborg, & C. Crumley (Eds.), *The world system and the earth system* (pp. 280–287). Left Coast Press.

Devezas, T. (2020). The struggle SARS-CoV-2 vs. Homo sapiens – Why the earth stood still, and how will it keep moving on? *Technological Forecasting and Social Change, 160*, 1–5. doi.org/10.1016/j.techfore.2020.120264. https://doi.org/10.1016/j.techfore.2020.120264

Eisenberg, M., & Mordechai, L. (2019). Rejecting catastrophe: The case of the Justinianic Plague. *Past & Present, 244*(1), 3–50. doi.org/10.1093/pastj/gtz009. https://doi.org/10.1093/pastj/gtz009

Gabuev, A. (2020, March 23). The pandemic could tighten China's grip on Eurasia. *Foreign Policy.com*

Genicot, L. (1966). Crisis: From the Middle Ages to Modern times. In M. M. Postan (Ed.), *The Cambridge economic history of Europe* (Vol. 1. 2nd ed., pp. 660–741). Cambridge University Press.

Gibbon, E. (1994). *The history of the decline and fall of the Roman Empire*. Allen Lane. (Original work published 1776)

Goldstone, J. (1991). *Revolution and rebellion in the early modern world*. University of California Press.

Harper, K. (2017). *The fate of Rome*. Princeton University Press.

Jack, A., & Staton, B. (2021, March 8). Teachers grapple with lost year of learning. *Financial Times*, 4.

Jacobs, E. (2020, November 2). Long Covid casts and enduring shadow over workers. *Financial Times*, 14.

Jones, P. (1966). Italy. In M. M. Postan (Ed.), *The Cambridge economic history of Europe* (Vol. 1. 2nd ed., pp. 340–431). Cambridge University Press.

Karatasli, S. S. (2020). Pandemic's lesson: Global capitalism is uneven and dangerously particularistic. Retrieved November 2, 2020, from http://chs.asa-comparative-historical.org/pandemics-lesson-global-capitalism-is-uneven-and-dangerously-particularistic/

Kohler, T., & Smith, M. (Eds.). (2018). *Ten thousand years of inequality: The archaeology of wealth differences*. University of Arizona Press.

Livi-Bacci, M. (2008). *Conquest: The destruction of the American Indios*. Polity.

Lopez, R. (1967). *The birth of Europe*. Evans and Company.

Maddicott, J. R. (1997). Plague in 7th century England. *Past and Present, 156*(1), 7–54. https://doi.org/10.1093/past/156.1.7

Mahbubani, K. (2020). After the coronavirus. *Foreign Policy, 236*(Spring), 9–13.

McCormick, M. (2001). *The origins of the European economy.* Cambridge University Press.

McMillen, C. (2016). *Pandemics: A very short introduction.* Oxford University Press.

McNeill, W. (1976). *Plagues and peoples.* Anchor Press.

Morris, I. (2010). *Why the West rules – for now.* Farrar, Straus, and Giroux.

Morris, I. (2013). *The measure of civilization.* Princeton University Press.

Morris, I. (2014, February 28). Plagues and economic collapse. *Darwin College Lecture Series.* Retrieved November 1, 2020, from https://sms.cam.ac.uk/media/1667998

Ostrogorsky, G. (1966). Agrarian conditions in the Byzantine Empire in the Middle Ages. In M. M. Postan (Ed.), *The Cambridge economic history of Europe* (Vol. 1. 2nd ed., pp. 205–234). Cambridge University Press.

Pearce-Duvet, J. (2006). The origin of human pathogens: Evaluating the role of agriculture and domestic animals in the evolution of human disease. *Biological Reviews, 81*(3), 369–382. https://doi.org/10.1017/S1464793106007020

Pennisi, E. (2018). A tropical parasitic disease has invaded Europe, thanks to a hybrid of two infectious worms. *Science Magazine.* Retrieved November 4, 2020, from https://www.sciencemag.org/news/2018/08/tropical-parasitic-disease-has-invaded-europe-thanks-hybrid-two-infectious-worms

Politi, J., & Fedor, L. (2020, September 4). US virtual schooling deals blow to recovery hopes. *Financial Times,* 3.

Postan, M. M. (1966). England. In M. M. Postan (Ed.), *The Cambridge economic history of Europe* (Vol. 1. 2nd ed., pp. 549–632). Cambridge University Press.

Rogers, T. (2021, June 8). America's small businesses get creative to attract workers. *Financial Times,* 3.

Roos, R. (2004, January 14). WHO sees more evidence of civet role in SARS. *Center for Infectious Disease Research and Policy.* Retrieved November 4, 2020, from https://www.cidrap.umn.edu/news-perspective/2004/01/who-sees-more-evidence-civet-role-sars

Russell, J. C. (1969). Population in Europe 500-1500. In C. Cipolla (Ed.), *The Fontana economic history of Europe: Vol. 1* (pp. 25–70). Collins/Fontana.

Schake, K. (2020). After the coronavirus. *Foreign Policy, 236*(Spring), 9–13.

Scheidel, W. (2017). *The great leveler: Violence and the history of inequality from the Stone Age to the twenty-first century.* Princeton University Press.

Smallman-Raynor, M. R., & Cliff, D. C. (2004). *War epidemics.* Oxford University Press.

Smith, R. (1966). Spain. In M. M. Postan (Ed.), *The Cambridge economic history of Europe* (Vol. 1. 2nd ed., pp. 432–448). Cambridge University Press.

Thucydides. (1974). *The Peloponnesian War* (Rex Warner, Trans.). Penguin. (Original work published c400 BCE/)

Trade, health and social reproduction in a COVID world

Silke Trommer 🆔

ABSTRACT
Building on feminist International Political Economy scholarship, my paper traces the effects of the COVID-19 pandemic on the trade and health nexus, taking into account the global productive economy and the realm of social reproduction. I argue that COVID-19 has exacerbated the socio-economic inequalities, including the crisis in social reproduction, that characterised the trade and health nexus prior to COVID-19. However, no ideational shift has taken place during the pandemic whereby trade policy communities conceive of trade as a tool for equitable and sustainable forms of social reproduction, as advocated by feminists, environmentalists, and others. This leaves the exploitative nature of global trade relations and their ambivalent relationship with health and social reproduction intact. I conclude that building back better from COVID-19 requires an ambitious redrawing of global trade relations and discuss a number of reforms that could be applied by global trade institutions today.

Introduction

COVID-19 and global trade are closely linked. The pandemic spreads across the world via the globally integrated trading system. It also unsettles global trade relations, prompting, among others, a collapse in trade flows (WTO, 2021a), and World Trade Organization (WTO)'s talks on the partial suspension of Intellectual Property (IP) protections in the Agreement on Trade-Related Aspects of Intellectual Property Rights (TRIPS), known as the 'TRIPS waiver' (WTO, 2021b). At the time of writing, commentators see the 'trade environment' as being 'in a state of flux' (World Economic Forum, 2021). With political tensions and uncertainty characterizing the trading system already prior to COVID-19 (McNamara et al., 2021; Scott & Wilkinson, 2021), the pandemic will likely alter global trade relations, although to what extent remains unclear.

My article contributes to reflections on how the pandemic might transform world trade by examining the effects of COVID-19 on the so-called trade and health nexus through a feminist International Political Economy (IPE) lens.

Global trade and human health are linked in ambivalent ways (Gleeson & Labonté, 2020). Trade helps producing welfare, knowledge and technology, which can benefit health (Feachem, 2001). Trade also acts as a vector for disease transmission and creates social and economic inequalities, which undermine health (Lee, 2000; Woodward et al., 2002). Legal rules in trade agreements can interfere with the availability and affordability of medical products, nutrition and food safety, health care services, and a clean environment, which are all essential for health (Barlow et al.,

2021). The trade and health nexus is explored across public health, international law, and IPE scholarship, yet few scholars take a feminist approach.

While there are many different feminisms, a feminist IPE lens centres social reproduction at the heart of the analysis of global trade relations (Hannah et al., 2021a). Social reproduction refers to 'the activities and attitudes, behaviors and emotions, and responsibilities and relationships directly involved in maintaining life on a daily basis and intergenerationally' (Brenner & Laslett, 1991, p. 314), or, in other words, 'all those activities involved in the production of life' (Elias & Rai, 2019, p. 203).

Social reproductive labour includes care work for children, the sick and the elderly, food provisioning, and other domestic and household chores necessary for daily life. According to feminist public health scholars, social reproduction aims to achieve or maintain human health (Elson, 2012), although social reproductive labour can be carried out under conditions that undermine health (Doyal, 1995). Feminist IPE criticizes that social reproductive work is generally unpaid or underpaid, and, where it takes place in domestic spheres, is not considered to be part of the quantified, productive economy, despite being essential for the productive economy to exist (Bakker, 2007; Griffin, 2007; Peterson, 2005). As Tithi Bhattacharya explains, the COVID-19 pandemic 'has clarified what social reproduction feminists have been saying for a while, which is that care work and life-making work are the essential work of society' (Jaffe, 2020; see also Mezzadri, 2020). The COVID-19 pandemic has reinforced social norms that attribute reproductive labour to women (UN Women & Women Count, 2020).

Below, I argue that a feminist IPE lens can recalibrate trade and health debates because it recognizes social reproduction and life- and health-making as essential economic activities. In consequence, the common subordination of health and life-making work to growth and profit-making work in global trade constitutes a form of economic inequality and exploitation. To assess how the pandemic might transform global trade, I ask how the COVID-19 trade collapse and the WTO TRIPS waiver affect the relationship between social reproduction, trade and health.

I find that trade policy-makers and observers have so far failed to meaningfully debate how global trade relations may support rather than exploit social reproduction, including life- and health-making activities. Instead, most commentators continue to conceptualize trade as a tool for generating growth within the productive economy, through which they hope ostensibly 'trade-related' policy goals, such as health, may be achieved (see also McNamara et al., 2021). They implicitly or explicitly accept that global trade in its current configuration supports good health and social reproductive conditions for some populations, while undermining health and social reproduction efforts of others. In the first years of the pandemic, the opportunity has been missed to head the demands of feminists, environmentalists and others that trade flows and practices must secure equitable and sustainable forms of producing and maintaining life on the planet for all (Gallogly-Swan & Brett, 2020; Hannah et al., 2021a; Klein, 2014; Orbie, 2020). I conclude that at the time of writing, social reproduction and health concerns are set to remain second-order issues in post-pandemic global trade relations, despite the fact that trade institutions could introduce many policy changes today that would alleviate the unequal effects of trade on social reproduction and health.

Social reproduction, trade and health

Prior to COVID-19, IPE works on trade and health focused on IP protections in Trade and Investment Agreements (TIA) and access to medicines (Hannah, 2016; Muzaka, 2011; Odell & Sell, 2006).

Public health and international legal scholarship exposes an exclusive IP focus as too narrow. As detailed below, trade rules and practise affect health via trade in goods, service and investment liberalization, food and safety standards, environmental and social provisions, and more (for a recent review see Gleeson & Labonté, 2020).

Furthermore, IPE analysis of global trade typically fails to systematically interrogate how trade relates to social reproduction. Most scholarship carries conceptual blindspots, whereby 'the economy' refers to the productive economy, while social reproduction remains invisible and undervalued as an economic sphere (Prügl, 2020). How trade rules and practices affect unpaid care work, domestic work, and social reproductive conditions is obscured and under-researched. Only recently has feminist IPE of trade scholarship begun drawing systematic attention to how trade affects social reproduction (Hannah et al., 2018; Roberts et al., 2019).

I argue that trade and health debates can learn from feminist insights that social reproduction is not only occupied with life- and health-making, as feminist health scholars assert, but that life- and health-making are economic activities, even when carried out within domestic or household settings, as feminist IPE stresses. Standard conceptualizations of health as a second order issue in trade policy (for a recent critique see van Schalwyk et al., 2021) do not stand up to feminist scrutiny. If formal and informal, paid and unpaid social reproductive labour that works to maintain life and health is economic in nature, then how trade rules and practices affect life- and health-making are central trade issues, and not second-order, trade-related issues. Gendered hierarchies of what is valuable economic activity are part of the 'norms of the international trading system' that public health scholars believe to 'obscure the interdependence between trade and health and […] impede states' abilities to enact structural changes for equitable health and economic systems' (Yang et al., 2020, p. 1).

The burdens that trade rules and practices place on health and life-making are one dimension of capitalism's exploitative relationship with social reproduction (Fraser, 2016; Mezzadri, 2020). Feminists argue that the pursuit of economic growth and capitalist accumulation tend to destabilize social reproduction. Historically, capitalist society de-values social reproduction and casts it into the 'private' domain. Today, falling wages and public funding cuts increasingly commodify and stretch thin social reproduction (Fraser, 2016). Trade rules and practices that affect the availability and affordability of medical products, healthy foods, care services, and a clean environment via goods, service and investment liberalization, food and safety standards, environmental and social provisions are one mechanism of this larger trend.

In response, feminist IPE of trade scholars ask for trade policies and practices to support progressive forms of social reproduction, rather than supporting economic growth and profit within the productive economy (Hannah et al., 2021a, 2021b). They demand that trade scholars and practitioners take into account not only how trade affects state actors, businesses and investors, but also citizens in their roles as workers, carers, consumers, unpaid labourers, and people expending leisure time (Roberts et al., 2019). In trade and health debates, supporting progressive forms of social reproduction means forging trade relations that enable good health and care conditions for all of these groups, everywhere. As discussed below, the COVID-19 trade collapse and the WTO TRIPS waiver are unlikely to generate such transformations.

Social reproduction, health and the COVID-19 trade collapse

In 'the steepest [dip] on record' (WTO, 2020a), global merchandise trade dropped by 18.5% in the second quarter of 2020 compared to the second quarter of 2019. In service trade, sectors relying on physical proximity between the buyer and seller (e.g. tourism, transport) were hit hardest, while sectors trading online were better shielded from the economic impact of the pandemic (e.g. finance and insurance) or benefitted (e.g. online retail) (Shingal, 2020). While global merchandise trade is expected to increase by 8% in 2021 and 4% in 2022, the recovery is highly uneven and in part contingent on the global vaccination roll-out (WTO, 2021c).

The COVID-19 trade collapse is largely a collapse of globalized production and global food systems. Since approximately the 1980s, global trade increasingly occurs in intermediary products and services. Today, complex production networks controlled by corporations and investors provide most things we consume daily (Linsi, 2020). These global productive configurations accelerated the global spread of COVID-19. When outbreaks and public health measures slowed down production in various regions of the world, economic shocks travelled along transnational production chains to affect the global productive economy as a whole (Baldwin, 2020; Linsi, 2020).

The COVID-19 trade collapse puts pressure on social reproduction. Public health scholars anticipate that pandemic-induced 'changes to the global trading landscape have wide-ranging consequences for physical and mental health, as they affect supplies of drugs and medical equipment, nutrition and food security, and government income necessary to pay for health services' (Barlow et al., 2021, e102). As public services become stretched, the COVID-19 trade collapse pushes care work out of the productive economy and into domestic settings. The increased scarcity of products essential for social reproduction, such as medical products and food, further increases the economic burden on health and life-making activities. Feminists emphasize that these types of trade adjustments typically disproportionately affect women and other vulnerable populations, who are primarily responsible for social reproductive labour, while lacking the economic, social and political resources to absorb trade shocks (Hannah et al., 2018; Roberts et al., 2019; van Staveren et al., 2007). Thus, the social reproductive crises inherent in the COVID-19 trade collapse do not occur evenly across the global economy, but particularly afflict already marginalized groups.

These mechanisms perpetuate the uneven relationship between trade, health and social reproduction that pre-dates COVID-19, whereby participation in global trade supports good social reproductive and health conditions for some populations, while other populations' health and social reproductive processes are undermined. Public health scholarship arguably provides evidence for this view, when it theorizes the links between trade adjustments and health outcomes based on the widely accepted notion that trade liberalization always creates winners and losers (Blouin et al., 2009). Public health scholars link shifts in income distribution and economic inequality and insecurity resulting from trade policy change to shifts in mortality (Blouin et al., 2009; McNamara, 2017). They also provide detailed accounts of how trade adjustments negatively affect the conditions in which people live, learn, work, and play, which can have detrimental effects on health, including mental health (Corrigall et al., 2008; Labonté et al., 2007; McNamara, 2017). From a feminist IPE perspective, these mechanisms constitute trade-induced crises of social reproduction. They result, in part, from sets of global trade relations that pay limited attention to how trade affects life- and health-making beyond the realm of the productive economy.

The links between trade, health and social reproduction do not receive full attention in trade policy circles in the ongoing pandemic. Policy debates and initiatives focus on weaknesses in the global productive economy around key social reproductive products, notably pharmaceuticals, medical equipment, and food. At the start of the pandemic, more than 80 countries imposed export restrictions on social reproductive products (Baldwin & Evenett, 2020; Linsi, 2020). Some briefly advocated a debundling of global production networks in strategically relevant sectors (Betti & Hong, 2020; Vela, 2020). Given the scale of global economic interdependences, however, many favour trade policies that facilitate the transnational production of social reproductive items, such as tariff elimination, removal of export restrictions and facilitation of border checks (OECD, 2020), which are also seen as essential trade policy tools for a global economic recovery (Baldwin & Evenett, 2020).

Trade policy circles do not acknowledge the toll that global trade in its current configuration takes on health and life-making efforts of certain populations. Policy-makers design trade policy tools that support global production networks within the existing framework of trade rules and practices. These practices leave the exploitative relationship between trade, health, and social reproduction in global economic relations intact. For example, labour exploitation is on the rise, leading, among other things, to increased risks of COVID-19 infection and illness (European Union Agency for Fundamental Rights, 2020; Ratcliffe, 2021). Yet, there are no signs of renewed interest in trade policy circles in labour rights beyond references to the International Labour Organisation (ILO) Declaration in TIAs, which create no legally enforceable commitments on labour standards (McNamara et al., 2021). As discussed below, despite unprecedented talks on a WTO TRIPS waiver, trade policy circles do not appear to recognize that we need to fundamentally reformulate all trade relations, in order to directly tackle the health and reproductive crises that participation in world trade imposes on certain populations.

Social reproduction, health and the WTO TRIPS waiver

In October 2020, India and South Africa proposed a WTO waiver to suspend patents and other TRIPS provisions in relation to the prevention, containment and treatment of COVID-19 for the duration of the pandemic (WTO, 2020b). The proposal carves out policy space for governments to scale up manufacturing capacities of medicines, vaccines, diagnostics and other medical products essential to fight COVID-19. The European Union (EU), the United Kingdom (UK) and Norway, among others, believe that existing IPRs enable the effective development and supply of medical products. They point to the 2001 WTO Doha Declaration on TRIPS and Public Health that reconfirmed TRIPS flexibilities in the context of the global HIV/AIDS crisis (Abbott, 2002). The United States (US) backed the TRIPS waiver in May 2021, providing the political moment that may lead to the launch of text-based WTO negotiations in the second half of 2021 (WTO, 2021b).

Scholars, health activists and international agencies have long criticized IP protection in TIAs as negatively affecting the accessibility and affordability of medical products, which are essential for health and life-making in public and domestic care settings. They critique that the ability to use legal flexibilities is not evenly distributed across the global economy. Poor countries in particular typically lack the social transfer systems and the bureaucratic capacity to use TRIPS exceptions in order to make medical products affordable for their populations. Rigid IP protection in TIAs can also hinder efforts to supply affordable medicines during public health emergencies (Coriat et al., 2006; Cullet, 2003; Gleeson & Friel, 2013; Gleeson & Labonté, 2020; Médecins Sans Frontières, 2020; Musungu et al., 2006; Sell, 2007).

The TRIPS waiver by itself is unlikely to resolve these issues. First, the US so far only supports a patent waiver, while the original proposal tackles additional TRIPS clauses that shape the global distribution of medical products (Bosse et al., 2021). Second, many bilateral and regional TIAs go beyond TRIPS provisions, but are not covered under the waiver (McNamara et al., 2021). Third, the global IP regime anchored in TIAs is only one aspect of a wider set of trade and economic policies through which corporations, not states, govern global production networks (Hannah, Scott, et al., 2021). States and non-state actors may need to actively challenge power relations in global production, in order to force the equitable global distribution of products required to fight the pandemic.

The TRIPS waiver debate does not acknowledge how legal rules in TIAs link to health and social reproductive inequalities more widely. Public health and international legal scholars identify negative impacts of many standard clauses on the conditions for life- and health-making, with difficulties compounded in low- and middle-income countries (Charnovitz, 2000; Friel et al., 2014; Koivusalo, 2004; McNeill et al., 2017; Shaffer et al., 2005). Studies suggest that health and social services liberalization commitments in TIAs damage the equity and efficiency of health care systems (Jarman & Greer, 2010; Woodward, 2005). Investment protection provisions compound these effects by putting a costly tag on adjusting economic policies for public policy reasons if investors decide to take governments to investor-state arbitration for compensation of losses (Labonté et al., 2016). In the context of COVID-19, it is conceivable that investors sue governments over lockdown measures (Ranjan & Anand, 2020). Some voices have thus called for a moratorium on all investment arbitration in relation to the pandemic (Columbia Centre on Sustainable Investment Law, 2020). Rules applying to national food and agricultural safety law under Sanitary and Phytosanitary (SPS) provisions in TIAs may also prevent governments from seeking health protections, but do not incorporate minimum health standards, and lack clarity on the integration of scientific knowledge (including its limits) and the use of product labelling when balancing health and trade concerns (Charnovitz, 2000).

Legal provisions in TIAs create health and social reproductive inequalities by benefitting corporations providing healthcare products and services within the productive economy, but curtailing government intervention and spending in health and other areas relevant for social reproduction, such as social and environmental policy (Gleeson & Friel, 2013; McNamara et al., 2021). They are typically imposed even when they breach international legal commitments relating to social reproduction, such as the right to health and human, labour and environmental rights, although mutually supportive legal interpretations of commitments are often possible (Doumbia-Henry & Gravel, 2006; Forman, 2007; Harrison, 2007; Vranes, 2009). Where TIA provisions set out procedures to balance commercial interests and broader societal interests, they are typically interpreted in ways that benefit commercial interests (Charnovitz, 2000). TIA negotiations empower corporate actors and investors, representing e.g. unhealthy foods, alcohol and tobacco industries, private health, care and education providers, and pharmaceutical industries over health-policy makers, women's groups, or other interests linked to social reproduction (Friel et al., 2013; Hannah et al., 2021a; Labonté et al., 2011). Women and other vulnerable populations disproportionately suffer under the resulting social reproductive and health crises, as they do under adjustment shocks following changes in trade flows (Hannah et al., 2018; Roberts et al., 2019).

TIAs forged during the COVID-19 pandemic drive forward the so-called twenty-first-century trade agenda, including new rules on government procurement and e-commerce, which health scholars suspect may negatively impact life and health-making (McNamara et al., 2021). According to the WTO, 46 TIAs have been signed or entered into force in 2020 (WTO, 2020c, 2020d).[1] Despite civil society campaigns demanding a moratorium on trade talks during the pandemic (e.g. Friends of the Earth International, 2020), TIAs are rolled out on all continents. This includes the African Continental Free Trade Agreement, the Regional Comprehensive Economic Partnership in South-East Asia, South America's Mercosur negotiations with Canada, the European Free Trade Area, Singapore and South Korea, the UK-EU trade deal and the various UK post-Brexit TIAs, and the United States-Mexico-Canada Agreement.

No debate has emerged on how TIAs must be reformed so that global trade does not invariably create a social reproductive and health crisis somewhere in the global economy. Trade policy-makers and observers remain wedded to the idea that trade agreements are a tool for economic growth, which provides health and other social reproductive products and services via the productive economy. Trade law initiatives during the pandemic continue to undermine public policy infrastructures and policy space that support healthy and equitable modes of producing life on the planet.

Conclusion

The COVID-19 pandemic has upset global trade flows and brought important shifts in how policy-makers think about IP provisions in TIAs. A feminist IPE analysis finds little to suggest, however, that the COVID-19 crisis is leading trade policy-makers and commentators to think differently about the links between trade, health and social reproduction. Instead, they continue to see global trade relations as a tool for generating economic growth within the productive economy, although these processes engender health and social reproductive crises for certain populations. As long as we accept the ideas that the productive economy and social reproduction are separate spheres, and that trade relations always create winners and losers, trade and health debates continue to be reduced to the question: 'whose health and social reproductive conditions thrive and whose suffer under global trade?', rather than asking 'how can we forge global trade relations that foster good health and good social reproductive conditions for all?'

Meanwhile, some commentators have argued already before the pandemic that we must reorient trade policies to support progressive social and environmental goals, rather than supporting economic growth (Gallogly-Swan & Brett, 2020; Hannah et al., 2021a; Klein, 2014; Orbie, 2020). Findings in health scholarship that wealth distribution is the more important for health outcomes than economic growth (Blouin et al., 2009; Godziewski, 2020) and that health agendas must be cognizant of social inequalities such as gender (Davies et al., 2019) support calls for trade policies that work for equitable and sustainable modes of producing life on the planet.

The scholarship evoked throughout my article has made many detailed proposals for achieving progressive reforms of the trade and health nexus in the immediate term. While it is impossible to review all proposals here, changes that governments and trade institutions can make today include:

- Adopt the WTO TRIPS Waiver as originally proposed, extend flexibilities to bilateral and regional TIAs and work with non-state actors to challenge the power relations that uphold the unequal global distribution of products required to fight the pandemic.
- Impose a moratorium on trade negotiations and on investment arbitration and other clauses in TIAs that directly impact health and social reproductive products and services.
- Honour commitments towards health and social reproduction across all instruments of international law, including human rights, labour and environmental commitments.
- When interpreting TIA provisions, strike a balance between commercial interests and broader societal interests that put good health and social reproductive conditions first.

Broader efforts to shift our thinking about social reproduction, trade and health require a larger exercise of reflection and consultation among all groups who partake in global trade relations daily. This includes not only state agents, business representatives and investors, but also workers, consumers, carers, and citizens. It also includes those theorizing the links between trade and inequality and trade and environmental depletion. The biggest positive impact COVID-19 could have on global trade relations would be to bring such broader coalitions together, both in trade theory and in trade politics.

Note

1. At the time of writing no WTO data on new TIAs is available for 2021.

Disclosure statement

No potential conflict of interest was reported by the author(s).

Funding

This work was supported by the Social Sciences and Humanities Research Council of Canada (SSHRC) [grant number 430-2018-00349] and the SSHRC-Economic and Social Research Council Knowledge Synthesis [grant number 872-2018-0012].

ORCID

Silke Trommer ⓘ http://orcid.org/0000-0001-9719-8065

References

Abbott, F. (2002). The Doha declaration on the TRIPS agreement and public health: Lighting a dark corner at the WTO. *Journal of International Economic Law, 5*(2), 469–505. https://doi.org/10.1093/jiel/5.2.469

Bakker, I. (2007). Social reproduction and the constitution of a gendered political economy. *New Political Economy, 12*(4), 541–556. https://doi.org/10.1080/13563460701661561

Baldwin, R. (2020). The greater trade collapse of 2020: Learnings from the 2008–09 great trade collapse. Voxeu.org Column. https://voxeu.org/article/greater-trade-collapse-2020

Baldwin, R., & Evenett, S. (2020). *COVID-19 and trade policy: Why turning inward won't work.* Centre for Economic Policy Research.

Barlow, P., van Schalwyk, M., McKee, M., Labonté, R., & Stuckler, D. (2021). COVID-19 and the collapse of global trade: Building an effective public health response. *The Lancet Planetary Health, 5*(2), e102–e107. https://doi.org/10.1016/S2542-5196(20)30291-6

Betti, F., & Hong, P. (2020). *Coronavirus is disrupting global value chains: Here's how companies can respond.* World Economic Forum. https://www.weforum.org/agenda/2020/02/how-coronavirus-disrupts-global-value-chains/

Blouin, C., Chopra, M., & van der Hoeven, R. (2009). Trade and social determinants of health. *The Lancet, 373*(9662), 502–507. https://doi.org/10.1016/S0140-6736(08)61777-8

Bosse, J., Kang, H. Y., & Thambisetty, S. (2021, May 7). Trips waiver: There's more to the story than vaccine patents. *The Conversation.* Retrieved 25 June 25, 2021, from https://theconversation.com/trips-waiver-theres-more-to-the-story-than-vaccine-patents-160502

Brenner, J., & Laslett, B. (1991). Gender, social reproduction, and women's self-organization: Considering the U.S. welfare state. *Gender & Society, 5*(3), 311–333. https://doi.org/10.1177/089124391005003004

Charnovitz, S. (2000). The supervision of health and biosafety regulation by world trade rules. *Tulane Environmental Law Journal, 13*(2), 271–302.

Colombia Centre on Sustainable Investment Law. (2020). Calls for ISDS moratorium during COVID-19 crisis and response. http://ccsi.columbia.edu/2020/05/05/isds-moratorium-during-covid-19/

Coriat, B., Orsi, F., & d'Almeida, C. (2006). TRIPS and the international public health controversies: Issues and challenges. *Industrial and Corporate Change, 15*(6), 1033–1062. https://doi.org/10.1093/icc/dtl029

Corrigall, J., Plagerson, S., Lund, C., & Myers, J. (2008). Global trade and mental health. *Global Social Policy, 8*(3), 335–358. https://doi.org/10.1177/1468018108095632

Cullet, P. (2003). Patents and medicines: The relationship between TRIPS and the human right to health. *International Affairs, 79*(1), 139–160. https://doi.org/10.1111/1468-2346.00299

Davies, S., Harman, S., Manjoo, R., Tanyag, M., & Wenham, C. (2019). Why it must be a feminist global health agenda. *The Lancet, 393*(10171), 601–603. https://doi.org/10.1016/S0140-6736(18)32472-3

Doumbia-Henry, C., & Gravel, E. (2006). Free trade agreements and labour rights: Recent developments. *International Labour Review, 145*(3), 185–206. https://doi.org/10.1111/j.1564-913X.2006.tb00017.x

Doyal, L. (1995). *What makes women sick? Gender and the political economy of health.* Palgrave Macmillan.

Elias, J., & Rai, S. (2019). Feminist everyday political economy: Space, time, and violence. *Review of International Studies, 45*(2), 201–220. https://doi.org/10.1017/S0260210518000323

Elson, D. (2012). Social reproduction in the global crisis: Rapid recovery or long-lasting depletion? In P. Utting, S. Razavi, R. V. Buchholz, & R. Varghese Buchholz (Eds.), *The global crisis and transformative social change* (pp. 63–80). Palgrave Macmillan.

European Union Agency for Fundamental Rights. (2020). Stop labour exploitation and protect workers from COVID-19. https://fra.europa.eu/en/news/2020/stop-labour-exploitation-and-protect-workers-covid-19

Feachem, R. (2001). Globalisation is good for your health, mostly. *British Medical Journal, 323*(7311), 504–506. https://doi.org/10.1136/bmj.323.7311.504

Forman, L. (2007). Trade rules, intellectual property, and the right to health. *Ethics & International Affairs, 21*(3), 337–357. https://doi.org/10.1111/j.1747-7093.2007.000103.x

Fraser, N. (2016). Contradictions of capital and care. *New Left Review, 100,* 99–117.

Friel, S., Hattersley, L., Snowdon, W., Thow, A.-M., Lobstein, T., Sanders, D., Barquera, S., Mohan, S., Hawkes, C., Kelly, B., Kumanyika, S., L'Abbe, M., Lee, A., Ma, J., Macmullan, J., Monteiro, C., Neal, B., Rayner, M., Sacks, G., … Walker, C. (2013). Monitoring the impacts of trade agreements on food environments. *Obesity Reviews, 14,* 120–134. https://doi.org/10.1111/obr.12081

Friel, S., Hattersley, L., & Townsend, R. (2014). Trade policy and public health. *Annual Review of Public Health, 36*(1), 325–344. https://doi.org/10.1146/annurev-publhealth-031914-122739

Friends of the Earth International. (2020). Stop all trade and investment treaty negotiations during COVID-19 crisis and focus on access to medical supplies and saving lives: An open letter to trade ministries and the WTO. https://www.foei.org/news/letter-world-trade-organization-wto-covid19-coronavirus-medicine

Gallogly-Swan, K., & Brett, M. (2020). A climate retrofit: Next steps for UK trade. Manuscript on file with author.

Gleeson, D., & Friel, S. (2013). Emerging threats to public health from regional trade agreements. *The Lancet, 381*(9876), 1507–1509. https://doi.org/10.1016/S0140-6736(13)60312-8

Gleeson, D., & Labonté, R. (2020). *Trade agreements and public health: A primer for health policy makers, researchers and advocates.* Palgrave Macmillan.

Godziewski, C. (2020). As long as economic growth remains the EU's main objective, it will not be well prepared for health threats. *LSE European Politics and Policy (EUROPP) Blog.* https://blogs.lse.ac.uk/europpblog/2020/05/27/as-long-as-economic-growth-remains-the-eus-main-objective-it-will-not-be-well-prepared-for-health-threats/

Griffin, P. (2017). Refashioning IPE: What and how gender analysis teaches international (global) political economy. *Review of International Political Economy, 14*(4), 719–736. https://doi.org/10.1080/09692290701475437

Hannah, E. (2016). *NGOs and global trade: Non-state voices in EU policy-making.* Routledge.

Hannah, E., Roberts, A., & Trommer, S. (2018). *Gendering global trade governance through Canada-UK trade relations. Knowledge synthesis grant: Final report.* https://www.kings.uwo.ca/kings/assets/File/academics/polisci/bios/hannah/KSG-Final-Report.pdf

Hannah, E., Roberts, A., & Trommer, S. (2021a). Towards a feminist global trade politics. *Globalizations, 18*(1), 70–85. https://doi.org/10.1080/14747731.2020.1779966

Hannah, E., Roberts, A., & Trommer, S. (2021b). Gender in global trade: Transforming or reproducing trade orthodoxy? *Review of International Political Economy.* https://doi.org/10.1080/09692290.2021.1915846

Hannah, E., Scott, J., Trommer, S., & Harman, S. (2021). The global approach to vaccine equity is failing: additional steps that would help. Retrieved June 25, 2021, from https://theconversation.com/the-global-approach-to-vaccine-equity-is-failing-additional-steps-that-would-help-158711

Harrison, J. (2007). *The human rights impact of the world trade organisation*. Hart Publishing.

Jaffe, S. (2021, April 2). Social reproduction and the pandemic, with Tithi Bhattacharya. *Dissent Magazine*. Retrieved June 22, 2021, from https://www.dissentmagazine.org/online_articles/social-reproduction-and-the-pandemic-with-tithi-bhattacharya

Jarman, H., & Greer, S. (2010). Crossborder trade in health services: Lessons from the European laboratory. *Health Policy, 94*(2), 158–163. https://doi.org/10.1016/j.healthpol.2009.09.007

Klein, N. (2014). *This changes everything: Capitalism vs. the climate*. Penguin Books.

Koivusalo, M. (2014). Policy space for health and trade and investment agreements. *Health Promotion International, 29*(S1), i29–i47. https://doi.org/10.1093/heapro/dau033

Labonté, R., Blouin, C., & Chopra, M. (2007). *Towards health equitable globalization: Rights, regulation and redistribution*. Globalization knowledge network. Final report to the commission on social determinants of health. Institute of Population Health, University of Ottawa.

Labonté, R., Mohindra, K., & Lencucha, R. (2011). Framing international trade and chronic disease. *Globalization and Health, 7*(1), 21. https://doi.org/10.1186/1744-8603-7-21

Labonté, R., Schram, A., & Ruckert, A. (2016). The trans-pacific partnership: Is it everything we feared for in public health? *International Journal of Health Policy Management, 5*(8), 487–496. https://doi.org/10.15171/ijhpm.2016.41

Lee, K. (2000). The impact of globalization on public health: Implications for the UK faculty of public health medicine. *Journal of Public Health Medicine, 22*(3), 253–262. https://doi.org/10.1093/pubmed/22.3.253

Linsi, L. (2020). Speeding up slowbalization: Global value chains after COVID-19. In M. Campell-Verduyn, L. Linsi, S. Metinsoy, G. van Roozendaal, C. Egger, G. Fuller, & N. Voelkner (Eds.), *The COVID-19 pandemic: Continuity and change in the international political economy* (pp. 15–21). University of Groeningen and Globalisation Studies Groeningen.

McNamara, C. (2017). Trade liberalization and the social determinants of health: A state of the literature review. *Social Science & Medicine, 176*(3), 1–13. https://doi.org/10.1016/j.socscimed.2016.12.017

McNamara, C., Labonté, R., Schram, A., & Townsend, B. (2021). Glossary on free trade and health part 2: New trade rules and new urgencies in the context of COVID-19. *Journal of Epidemiology and Community Health, 75*(4), 407–412. https://doi.org/10.1136/jech-2020-215105

McNeill, D., Birkbeck, C., Fukuda-Parr, S., Grover, A., Schrecker, T., & Stuckler, D. (2017). Political origins of health inequities: Trade and investment agreements. *The Lancet, 389*(10070), 760–762. https://doi.org/10.1016/S0140-6736(16)31013-3

Mezzadri, A. (2020). A crisis like no other: Social reproduction and the regeneration of capitalist life during the COVID-19 pandemic. *Developing Economics Blog*. Retrieved June 22, 2021, from https://developingeconomics.org/2020/04/20/a-crisis-like-no-other-social-reproduction-and-the-regeneration-of-capitalist-life-during-the-covid-19-pandemic/

Médecins Sans Frontières. (2020). India and South Africa proposal for WTO waiver from intellectual property protections for COVID-19-related medical technologies. *Médecins Sans Frontières Briefing Document*. Retrieved November 30, 2020, from https://msfaccess.org/sites/default/files/2020-10/COVID_Brief_ProposalWTOWaiver_ENG_2020.pdf

Musungu, S., Oh, C., & World Health Organization. (2006). *The use of flexibilities in TRIPS by developing countries: Can they promote access to medicines?* South Centre.

Muzaka, V. (2011). *The politics of intellectual property rights and access to medicines*. Palgrave Macmillan.

Odell, J., & Sell, S. (2006). Reframing the issue: The WTO coalition on intellectual property and public health, 2001. In J. Odell (Ed.), *Negotiating trade: Developing countries in the WTO and NAFTA* (pp. 85–114). Cambridge University Press.

OECD. (2020). *COVID-19 and international trade: Issues and actions*.

Orbie, J. (2020). Freed from trade? Three steps towards a more progressive trade agenda. *UACES Network for EU-Africa Research Blog*. https://sites.google.com/view/network-of-eu-africa-research-/blog?authuser=0

Peterson, S. (2005). How (the meaning of) gender matters in political economy. *New Political Economy, 10*(4), 499–521. https://doi.org/10.1080/13563460500344468

Prügl, E. (2020). Untenable dichotomies: De-gendering political economy. *Review of International Political Economy*. https://doi.org/10.1080/09692290.2020.1830834

Ranjan, P., & Anand, P. (2020). COVID-19, India, and investor-state dispute settlement (ISDS): Will India be able to defend its public health measures? *Asia Pacific Law Review*. https://doi.org/10.1080/10192557.2020.1812255

Ratcliffe, R. (2021, June 13). Factory workers making goods for the west bear brunt of virus surge in South-East Asia. *The Guardian*.

Roberts, A., Trommer, S., & Hannah, E. (2019). Gender impacts of trade and investment agreements. Policy briefing prepared for the UK Women's Budget Group. https://wbg.org.uk/analysis/uk-policy-briefings/gender-impacts-of-trade-and-investment-agreements/

Scott, J., & Wilkinson, R. (2021). Reglobalizing trade: Progressive global governance in an age of uncertainty. *Globalizations*, *18*(1), 55–69. https://doi.org/10.1080/14747731.2020.1779965

Sell, S. (2007). TRIPS-plus free trade agreements and access to medicines. *Liverpool Law Review*, *28*(1), 41–75. https://doi.org/10.1007/s10991-007-9011-8

Shaffer, E., Waitzkin, H., & Brenner, J. (2005). Global trade and public health. *American Journal of Public Health*, *95*(1), 23–34. https://doi.org/10.2105/AJPH.2004.038091

Shingal, A. (2020). Services trade and COVID-9, Voxeu.or column. https://voxeu.org/article/services-trade-and-covid-19

UN Women & Women Count. (2020). Whose time to care? Unpaid care and domestic work during COVID-19. https://data.unwomen.org/publications/whose-time-care-unpaid-care-and-domestic-work-during-covid-19

van Schalwyk, M., Barlow, P., Siles-Brügge, G., Jarman, H., Hervey, T., & McKee, M. (2021). Brexit and trade policy: An analysis of the governance of UK trade policy and what it means for health and social justice. *Globalization and Health*. https://doi.org/10.1186/s12992-021-00697-1

van Staveren, I., Elson, D., Grown, C., & Çagatay, N. (2007). *The feminist economics of trade*. Routledge.

Vela, J. (2020). Coronavirus won't kill globalisation but it will clip its wings. *Politico*. https://www.politico.com/news/2020/04/22/coronavirus-europe-china-200333

Vranes, E. (2009). *Trade and the environment: Fundamental issues in international law, WTO law and legal theory*. Cambridge University Press.

Woodward, D. (2005). The GATS and trade in health services: Implications for health care in developing countries. *Review of International Political Economy*, *12*(3), 511–534. https://doi.org/10.1080/09692290500171021

Woodward, D., Drager, N., Beaglehole, R., & Lipson, D. (2002). *Globalization, global public goods and health*. Pan American Health Organization.

World Economic Forum. (2021). Global trade after COVID-19: From fixed capital to human capital. Retrieved June 22, 2021, from https://www.weforum.org/agenda/2021/05/the-global-trade-map-after-covid-19-from-fixed-capital-to-human-capital/

WTO. (2020a). Trade falls steeply in first half of 2020. Retrieved November 30, 2020, from https://www.wto.org/english/news_e/pres20_e/pr858_e.htm

WTO. (2020b). *Waiver from certain provisions of the TRIPS agreement for the prevention, containment and treatment of COVID-19: Communication from India and South Africa*. IP/C/W/669.

WTO. (2020c). Regional trade agreements database. Retrieved December 1, 2020, from https://rtais.wto.org/UI/PublicMaintainRTAHome.aspx

WTO. (2020d). *List of RTAs which have appeared in factual presentations (issued up to 6 November 2020) and have not yet been notified to the WTO*. WT/REG/W/154. WTO.

WTO. (2021a). COVID-19 and world trade. Retrieved June 22, 2021, from https://www.wto.org/english/tratop_e/covid19_e/covid19_e.htm

WTO. (2021b). Members approach text-based discussions for an urgent IP response to COVID-19. Retrieved June 22, 2021, from https://www.wto.org/english/news_e/news21_e/trip_09jun21_e.htm

WTO. (2021c). World trade primed for strong but uneven recovery after COVID 19 pandemic shock. Retrieved June 22, 2021, from https://www.wto.org/english/news_e/pres21_e/pr876_e.htm

Yang, J., Kotzias, V., Crosbie, E., & Mackey, T. (2020). COVID-19 and a window of opportunity: Guiding principles for a health-promoting trade agenda. *International Journal of Health Policy and Management*. https://doi.org/10.34172/IJHPM.2020.241

Shared pretenses for collective inaction: the economic growth imperative, COVID-19, and climate change

Diana Stuart ⓘ, Brian Petersen ⓘ and Ryan Gunderson ⓘ

ABSTRACT

This paper examines how the economic growth imperative not only drives climate change and created the conditions for the development and spread of the COVID-19 pandemic but is also the context for climate change inaction and ineffective responses to the pandemic. Focusing on the United States, the paper identifies pretenses for collective inaction on COVID-19 that are similar in content to familiar justifications for delay in climate action: (1) denialism, (2) individualism, and (3) techno-optimism. These justifications must be identified as strategies to maintain the status-quo and benefit the wealthy few while allowing avoidable human suffering and loss. Adequately addressing climate change and future pandemics requires overcoming these false narratives and transitioning to social conditions that are resilient, healthy, and sustainable – specifically conditions where social and ecological well-being are prioritized over economic growth for the sake of profit maximization.

Introduction

This manuscript examines similarities between the fractured and ineffective responses to COVID-19 in the United States (US) and the causes of climate 'inaction' or 'delay.' Responses to the pandemic, especially in the US, brings into clear sight the ongoing prioritization of *economic growth* before well-being, or profit before people and the environment. Economic growth refers to increasing levels of production, consumption, and wealth accumulation associated with increasing Gross Domestic Product (GDP). The 'growth imperative' refers to the prioritization of economic growth and a rejection of policies that slow growth, a priority built on the structural dynamics of capitalism. According to the growth imperative, growth is always good and must always be maintained. We focus on the US as an ideal case study. While all forms of capitalism require constant growth if they are to avoid the negative social impacts of unplanned recessions, as argued below, the form of neoliberal capitalism dominant in the US is especially prone to subordinating social and ecological wellbeing to economic growth and to 'fixat[e] on high GDP-growth-rates' (Ott, 2018, p. 7). This social context has had important implications for climate politics, including climate denial (see below). We argue this same social context provided an ideal breeding ground for COVID-19 inaction and justifications for delay.

Focusing on the US, where the growth imperative remains especially hegemonic, we examine how this imperative influenced the development and spread of COVID-19, drives climate change and, importantly here, steers policy responses to both. While other nations also consider impacts on economic growth in policy-making, the US context reveals what kinds of social outcomes emerge when the growth imperative remains a clear priority. In addition, in the US there remains a strong resistance to government intervention or 'big government,' even when intervention is necessary to minimize the impacts of a global pandemic as well as the climate crisis. We also focus much of our discussion on the Trump administration, whose blatant prioritization of wealth accumulation over climate stability and public health make this a compelling case to illuminate the justifications used to maintain the growth imperative.

With a focus on the US context, we identify three overlapping 'pretenses for inaction' between the slow and ineffective response to the pandemic and climate inaction: denialism, individualism, and techno-optimism. While we focus on discursive justifications for COVID-19 and climate inaction, we also shed light on the underlying social drivers of inaction through an analysis of how the growth imperative is built into the capitalist system. Societies find themselves in a paradoxical gridlock: the structural necessity to constantly expand growth is creating and maintaining forces that could undermine the prerequisites for growth and long-term human survival. The normative argument is that prioritizing growth hinders us from effectively addressing both climate change and a global pandemic.

The dual threats of COVID-19 and climate change bring a number of important questions to the fore (Cohen, 2020; Manzanedo & Manning, 2020; Newell & Dale, 2020; Robertson, 2020; Rosenbloom & Markard, 2020; Ruiu et al., 2020; Sarkis et al., 2020; Spash, 2020b; Yun, 2020). What impacts will the pandemic have on climate change responses and carbon emissions? What can we learn from responses to the COVID-19 pandemic for addressing climate change? Will COVID-19 serve as a climate crisis wake-up call, as a harbinger to transition to a more sustainable society? Although both global threats are 'invisible,' there is a marked difference between COVID-19 being widely regarded as an immediate threat that requires urgent, global action, while climate change is often (misleadingly) framed as a merely future-oriented risk and responses lack priority and urgency (Ruiu et al., 2020). While both crises pose serious threats to global populations, especially those who are already marginalized, the impacts of the climate crisis will be far greater and time to effectively and justly address climate change is running out (Markard & Rosenbloom, 2020).

While the COVID-19 crisis and the climate crisis are different along many lines (Fuentes et al., 2020), there are lessons we can learn through examining these crises together. First, their origin stories reveal a pattern of human domination over nature in a socioeconomic system that requires continually increasing material and energy throughput. Further, justifications for climate inaction and COVID-19 inaction overlap along at least three lines: (1) the denial of science, (2) a focus on inadequate individualized solutions, and (3) support for techno-fixes without social reforms. In both cases, these justifications were and continue to be used to support decisions that prioritize economic growth over human lives. This strategy protects the interests of the wealthy few, who benefit the most from a growth-oriented capitalist system (Oxfam, 2018), at the expense of those who are already most vulnerable and social and ecological well-being in general. We examine the similarities between these crises and why solutions that maintain the economic growth imperative will result in more loss and suffering that could be avoided. Identifying and overcoming false narratives (Wright, 2010) is a critical step to create the social conditions necessary to minimize the impacts of global warming and future pandemics.

The growth imperative, climate change, and the COVID-19 pandemic

To understand the inadequate responses to climate and COVID-19 crises, we must understand the role of the economic growth imperative. Here we use the term 'growth imperative' to refer to the structural necessity of capitalism to constantly increase production and consumption in order to accumulate capital. Before it was institutionalized as economic theory or policy goal, the growth imperative was already an underlying necessity of capitalist societies, 'rooted in capitalism's core competitive logic – the drive for profit and capital accumulation' (Antonio, 2013, p. 20). Capital has a structural necessity to self-expand and is, thus, growth dependent. As Speth (2008, p. 59) states, 'the capitalist economy, to the degree that it is successful, is inherently an exponential growth economy.' Along with competition, where firms must constantly reinvest profits to decrease costs and increase output, capitalist growth dependency is also driven by a pattern of lending, debt, investments in mass production infrastructure, and the necessary advertising to get consumers to purchase mass produced and excess goods (Blackwater, 2015).

Although it is now naturalized and common-sense that 'growth is good,' it was not until around the end of the Second World War that the growth imperative was institutionalized as an explicit aim of economic and social policy and became an organizing normative goal of economics (see Antonio, 2009; Schnaiberg, 1980). Ironically, GDP was used to measure productive capacity for the war effort and even the measurements creator, Simon Kuznets, stated it was not an appropriate indicator to assess well-being (Semuels, 2016). Yet, increasing annual GDP was widely adopted as a global economic and policy goal. That means every year more and more goods are produced and services offered. While some argue we need this growth to provide for a growing population, we are producing more and more per capita: global material production has quadrupled since 1970, growing twice as fast as the human population (Circle Economy, 2020).

During the mid-twentieth century 'Golden Age' of capitalism, growth was regulated and escalated by Keynesian welfare state policies. Following the financial crises and stagflation in the 1970s (Harvey, 2005), neoliberalism arose as an alternative growth regime, pushing tax cuts, austerity, and 'free markets' as new growth engines (Antonio, 2013). Despite the marked differences between Keynesian capitalism and neoliberal capitalism, both are bound to what Hamilton (2004) calls a 'growth fetish.' Mainstream economics views 'increasing affluence … as essentially equivalent to human well-being' (Dietz, 2015, p. 125).

Concerns with the ecological and social impacts of the growth imperative have mounted for decades. Ecological objections to the growth imperative were a cornerstone of early ecological economists (e.g. Daly, 1973; Georgescu-Roegen, 1971). Because economic growth requires increases in material and energy throughput, an economic system that is growth dependent is not ecologically sustainable (Schnaiberg, 1980). Economic growth is associated with increases in carbon emissions, national ecological footprints, and other environmental pressures, and an absolute decoupling of environmental impacts from economic growth at the rate necessary to avoid surpassing global warming targets is infeasible (for reviews, see Hickel & Kallis, 2020; Parrique et al., 2019; Schor & Jorgenson, 2019). Without evidence that decoupling at the rate necessary is possible, a reliance on the idea of green growth remains a risky gamble with vast moral implications (Stuart et al., 2020a).

Prioritizing economic growth has also been criticized on social grounds. Growth has failed to improve happiness after a relatively low level of development or alleviate global poverty, and has resulted in staggering levels of inequality (Hickel, 2017). The financial gains from GDP growth largely go to the wealthiest: in 2018 the world's richest 1% received 82% of global wealth (Oxfam,

2018). A growing number of economists, including Joseph Stiglitz (2009, 2019), continue to argue that GDP growth should be abandoned as a social goal (see Dietz, 2015). One of the social problems created by growth-dependency is vulnerability to negative growth: the inability of growth-dependent societies to resiliently respond to reductions in growth. In the growth-dependent society of global capitalism, 'nearly everyone … [is] dependent on growth whether it be through employment, financial investments, small business ownership, job security, retirement and health benefits, or life-style' (Antonio, 2009, p. 4; see Schnaiberg, 1980). In this context, reductions in growth (recessions and depressions) bring about social crises and harm. As detailed below, this second problem is especially clear in the case of the COVID-19 pandemic: '[t]he pandemic lockdowns serve to underscore once again that when economic growth comes to a halt, this economic system immediately enters a state of crisis' (Koch & Buch-Hansen, 2020).

The causes of the climate crisis and the COVID-19 pandemic cannot be understood outside of this political-economic context. Both crises can be traced to humans altering nature, including biophysical cycles, land use, and interactions with other species. The extraction and combustion of fossil fuels to support an energy-intensive and expanding economy, as well as high-carbon lifestyles (Urry, 2011), has resulted in a dramatic alteration of the carbon cycle (Intergovernmental Panel on Climate Change [IPCC], 2018). As some projections indicate 4°C of warming by 2100, depending on political choices made now, this crisis poses an existential threat. Leading scientists state that we cannot stay within climate targets without *rapid and radical* changes in *all* aspects of society (IPCC, 2018). Others have specifically pointed to economic growth as a major driver of both climate change and biodiversity loss. The alliance of world scientists (Ripple et al., 2020) state that: '[o]ur goals need to shift from GDP growth and the pursuit of affluence toward sustaining ecosystems and improving human well-being.' Similarly, Steffen et al. (2018, pp. 5–6) state that we need to change '[t]he present dominant socioeconomic system … based on high-carbon economic growth and exploitative resource use.' Others empirically illustrate that it is unlikely to impossible to keep global warming within 2°C in a growing economy (e.g. Hickel & Kallis, 2020; Parrique et al., 2019).

Like climate change, the COVID-19 pandemic is an outcome of human-nature interactions conditioned by a growth-dependent capitalist economy (Bhattacharya & Dale, 2020; Dale, 2020; Modonesi, 2020; Pazaitis et al., 2020; Spash, 2020b). While disease outbreaks preceded and will proceed capitalism, the causes and spread of the COVID-19 pandemic has a specific political-economic context. In terms of cause, zoonotic diseases proliferate in the current era, conditioned by the 'expansion of corporate agri-systems, encroachment of humans on habitats, and the commodification of wildlife – all integral to current growth economies' (Pazaitis et al., 2020, p. 614). The disease likely emerged from interactions with wildlife in Wuhan, China, and experts explain how these interactions resulted from climate change and habitat loss bringing humans and wildlife closer together as well as the transport of exotic mammals for human consumption (Dale, 2020). Further, the rapid pace by which the virus spread globally is unthinkable without an economically globalized world (Pazaitis et al., 2020). These altered socio-ecological relationships resulted in millions of deaths, and more pandemics will likely emerge as these altered relationships continue. In short, neither climate change nor COVID-19 are 'natural' (Dale, 2020), as both were caused by humans and the priorities that continue to drive humans to reshape the biophysical world. For both climate change and the COVID-19 pandemic, the underlying driver of these altered biophysical relationships is profit-oriented resource use, to support an ever-accelerating production-consumption engine.

Along with the causes of the dual crises, the growth imperative also shapes social responses to climate change and the COVID-19 pandemic. In capitalist societies, 'the economy' is a semi-autonomous system that dominates real human subjects and ecosystems for the abstract aim of capital accumulation. In these conditions, 'the bottom line' dominates trade-offs in sustainability discourse (Clark et al., 2018) as well as the pandemic (Bhattacharya & Dale, 2020; Spash, 2020b). The growth imperative not only drives us deeper into multiple crises, it also undermines the effectiveness of potential solutions. COVID-19 could have been addressed much more rapidly and effectively if governments were willing to quickly prioritize health and well-being. Similarly, we could have ended fossil-fuel use years ago and transformed our social systems to address climate change and prioritize social and ecological well-being. Each case reveals that much is lost when economic growth is prioritized.

While evidence illustrating the incompatibility of economic growth and climate change mitigation mount, the same trade-offs are clearer and easier to see through the faster-paced impacts of the COVID-19 pandemic. As Spash (2020b, p. 2) explains,

> [t]he coronavirus pandemic of 2020 provides a dramatic example of how modern economic systems are precariously structured to achieve financial returns. … [T]he primary capital accumulating motive, encapsulated in the economic growth imperative, means an inability of the system to pause even for a week, let alone a month or two, without economic and social crisis.

Debates early on focused on whether responses should prioritize the economy or public health. With lockdowns, we could avoid infection, but the production-consumption engine would dramatically slow down. In a society in which all livelihoods, through wages or profits, depend on the constant accumulation of capital, lockdowns without social safety nets prove disastrous for many. In the US, conservatives pushed for, and continue to push for, re-opening the economy before public health officials recommended. For example, representative Hollingsworth, the 12th wealthiest member of Congress, openly stated that the government should prioritize the economy and the American 'way of life' over minimizing the 'loss of life.' Hollingsworth was not alone in this view, as many states with conservative governors reopened early, with rising cases quickly following. Despite having the greatest number of cases and deaths globally, in late 2020 President Trump claimed positively that compared to other nations the US had 'experienced the smallest economic contraction,' explaining that 'a national lockdown costs $50 billion a day … this administration will not be going to a lockdown' (Trump Whitehouse Archives, 2020a).

President Trump and Republican governors' positions on lockdown and protective measures went against public opinion. In spring 2020, a *USA Today* poll showed that 72% of Americans believed we should prioritize public health, saving lives, and fighting Covid-19 over economic concerns (Shannon, 2020). Still, no national programme or plan to protect lives was implemented in the US during the Trump administration. At the same time, some politicians, pharmaceuticals companies, financers, and others view the pandemic as a 'great investment opportunity,' as put by the US Secretary of the Treasury, Steve Mnuchin (Carr, 2020).

The US was not the only country debating whether to prioritize the economy *or* public health. Despite diverse state responses to COVID-19, one consistency across the world is the push 'to accumulate with minimal sacrifice to profit' (Bhattacharya & Dale, 2020). In an international comparison of policy tools used by governments to respond to the pandemic, Capano et al. (2020, p. 295) found that 'the most commonly deployed government tools were economic in nature and the single most prevalent government responses in the dataset focused not on public health, per se, but rather on tax policy treatments to offset economic damage.' A 'herd immunity' strategy was considered by multiple countries at various times during the pandemic. As explained by Spash (2020b), the UK government considered a heard immunity strategy early on yet abandoned the idea when fatality rates were much higher than previously believed. Still, protective measures and testing was delayed in the UK. Sweden adopted an approach that kept businesses and schools open while encouraging protective measures. This resulted in a surge in cases and deaths compared to other Scandinavian countries, while failing to achieve herd immunity (Henley, 2020). While national responses to the pandemic greatly varied, these few examples illustrate that US leaders were not the only ones greatly concerned about economic growth. We focus here on the US, but acknowledge the more diverse global context.

The US, despite its immense resources, became the centre of global attention in 2020 as COVID-19 rates spiked dramatically. A herd immunity approach was discussed by US leaders as way to get the economy running at full speed, although Trump's hands-off approach was already resulting in the most cases worldwide. With 33 million cases and counting, the US is a particularly tragic example: delay, lack of testing, and lack of protective measures have resulted in an estimated 587, 245 deaths as of May 19, 2021 – *more than any other nation* and twice as many deaths as in India (John Hopkins Coronavirus Resource Center, 2021).

This section examined how the growth imperative drives carbon emissions and climate inaction as well as shaped the emergence of, and responses to, the COVID-19 pandemic. The following section expands this analysis by identifying overlapping justifications for ineffective responses to climate change and the COVID-19 pandemic, which we term 'pretenses for collective inaction.' As explained above, the push to 'save the economy' is an underlying pretense for collective inaction. The three shared pretenses for collective inaction detailed below – denial, individualism, and techno-optimism – are all derivative of the growth imperative necessitated by capital accumulation. Each justification is used to protect the growth imperative and those who continue to benefit the most from it. To illustrate these justifications, we draw from a diversity of publications from newspapers, magazines, Whitehouse Archives, and scholarly literature. The literature search specific to the COVID-19 pandemic was conducted in early 2021, thus most examples are specific to 2020. Examples were identified specifically because they illustrate the pretenses for collective inaction.

Shared pretenses for collective inaction

This section identifies three overlapping pretenses for inaction in climate politics and COVID-19 responses. Many countries ignored the World Health Organization's (WHO's) recommendation that countries prepare for the pandemic on February 11th, 2020 (Horta-Barba et al., 2020). However, there are stark differences between governments in policy responses and success in controlling the spread (Capano et al., 2020). We focus on the response in the US, which, along with Sweden, illustrated a 'less successful' policy response (Capano et al., 2020). Similarly, the US is one of the only countries to, until recently, pull out of the Paris Agreement and has relatively high levels of climate denialism. More broadly, the US offers an ideal case study for reasons explained in the introduction, namely the dominance of neoliberal ideology.

In comparison to explanations for climate inaction, which are increasingly refined in the social sciences (e.g. Blühdorn, 2007; Brulle & Norgaard, 2019; Ollinaho, 2016; Stoner & Melathopoulos, 2015), explanations for COVID-19 inaction are sparser. Some culprits for COVID-19 inaction include a 'massive, generalized bystander effect' at a global level (Horta-Barba et al., 2020, p. 915) and, specific to the US, federalism (Rocco et al., 2020), anti-rationality (Meeker, 2020), a lack of science literacy (Miller, 2020), and, as discussed below, individualism (Bazzi et al., 2020; Eichengreen, 2020). Here we shine light on overlapping justifications and pretenses for a lack of collective action to address climate change and the pandemic. In other words, we examine justifications for *not* implementing collective actions in response to both crises. Three shared pretenses for inaction are explored: denialism, individualism, and techno-optimism. As explained below, these three pretenses for inaction have been central to climate delay and were then echoed in justifications for failures to collectively address COVID-19. Denialism, individualism, and techno-optimism are pervasive, at least in part, because they overlook and leave untouched the system that not only drives climate change and the COVID-19 pandemic, but also its need to subordinate ecological well-being and public health to the growth imperative.

Denial as a shared pretense for collective inaction

Denialism is the first and clearest pretense for collective inaction common in climate politics and responses to COVID-19. Climate change denial and misinformation campaigns have been widely acknowledged, as well as their effectiveness in delaying climate policy (e.g. see Dunlap & Brulle, 2015). The clearest form of denial involves the outright rejection that anthropogenic climate change as a phenomenon exists. This outright denial was propagated widely by a well-organized and well-funded denial campaign. The fossil-fuel funded endeavour manufactured controversy about climate science, confused the public, and helped to thwart the ratification of the Kyoto Protocol. Tactics used included the use of fake experts, cherry-picking data, misrepresentation, logical fallacies, and conspiracy creation.

Another major form of denial is climate skepticism, which questions the credibility of science and the evidence supporting the need to act on climate change (Giddens, 2009). These typically involve economic or technical reasons to refute the science indicating that climate mitigation efforts are necessary and justifiable. Relatedly, neo-skepticism acknowledges the scientific basis for the climate crisis but denies the need to act in aggressive, proactive ways (Stern et al., 2016). Lastly, we see the rise of 'ideological denial' (Petersen et al., 2019): even people who acknowledge the climate crisis sometimes misdiagnose the drivers and promote inadequate and partial solutions that maintain the status quo. Mann (2021) identifies a shift from explicit, literal climate denialism to subtler forms of deflection like blaming individual consumers for emissions and promoting 'non-solution solutions' such as geoengineering. These trends are one of the threads connecting explicit denialism to individualism and techno-optimism as pretenses for inaction, discussed below.

With the election of President Trump in the US, there was a revival and surge in outright climate denial, denial that many believed had been largely put to rest by a 'unanimous' scientific consensus (Worland, 2017). Trump selected climate deniers and fossil fuel executives for key positions and maintained his position of dismissing climate change – having formerly called it a 'hoax' – while his administration dismantled climate initiatives in federal agencies (Worland, 2017) and withdrew the US from the Paris Agreement, claiming that it 'handicaps the US economy' and staying on would 'undermine our economy' (Trump White House Archives, 2017). The Trump administration has been widely cited for accelerating global warming and causing long-lasting and irreversible environmental harm (Popovich et al., 2021).

There are also different forms of COVID-19 denial, ranging from 'explicit' denial (e.g. calling COVID-19 a 'hoax,' as did former President Donald Trump) to 'implicit' denial (e.g. reopening 'the economy' before containing an outbreak) (Falkenbach & Greer, 2020). When the COVID-19 virus first emerged in Wuhan, China, there was a delayed response due to denial and suppression of information. In late December 2019, a Wuhan doctor shared that a SARS-like illness had been diagnosed among patients from a seafood market. This doctor and others who gave warnings were silenced by authorities and accused of spreading rumours. Reporters later revealed that this suppression was likely done to protect plans for an important government meeting of provincial leaders in Wuhan in mid-January 2020. When a team found evidence that the virus was transmittable from human to human, their findings were suppressed to avoid any panic that might disrupt the meeting. The government maintained that there were no new cases. Yet, by January 20th hundreds were infected. As the virus spread internationally, other governments and health agencies also denied the severity of the outbreak, spread misinformation, and chose to prioritize other goals before public health. The World Health Organization (WHO) was criticized for initially sharing the Chinese propaganda that the virus could not be spread through human-to-human transmission. The WHO also delayed calling the virus a pandemic until March, after there were cases in hundreds of countries. In trying to understand this misinformation and delay, political analysts highlighted the powerful donors who support the WHO and the political and economic pressures the organization faces.

In the US, the Trump administration downplayed and minimized the pandemic, spread blatant misinformation, and withheld resources for testing. Even the US Center for Disease Control (CDC) made false claims that COVID-19 could not be spread by asymptomatic individuals and that asymptomatic individuals should not be tested (Hauck, 2020). As with climate change, a nationally organized response to COVID-19 in the US was absent. Instead, public health experts and scientists were ignored and even attacked in order to prioritize economic concerns. At one point, the White House ordered hospitals to stop sending COVID-19 data to the CDC (Roston, 2020). *Time* magazine, called Trump a 'super-spreader of COVID misinformation' as he refused to wear a mask, told citizens not to be concerned about the pandemic, and stated that only weak people die from it (Bergengruen & Hennigan, 2020). Social media also played a significant role in amplifying the spread of misinformation.

Climate change denialism is most prevalent among conservatives (Dunlap et al., 2016). Similarly, COVID-19 denial is more common among conservatives and perpetuated by right-wing 'populist' politicians and governments (Falkenbach & Greer, 2020). Agius et al. (2020) argue that climate denial and COVID-19 denial are both marked by a nationalist and 'gendered' dimension. They are common among right-wing populists because the latter ideology is a reaction to an anxiety that one's security and identity are under threat ('ontological insecurity'). It is important to note that, in a growth-dependent economy, lockdowns and COVID-19-related unemployment without welfare provisions are, in fact, a threat to one's 'ontological security.' The lockdown protests can only be understood in this political-economic context (Burgis, 2020) in the same way that opposition to climate policy that does not have extensive job replacement provisions is understandable among those who work in carbon-intensive industries.

In both cases, there is a pattern of suppressing, ignoring, or refuting any science that might suggest solutions to protect people that happen to threaten economic growth and profits for powerful vested interests. A parallel 'attack on science' in the case of climate change and the pandemic was discussed in the media and among scientists, as very similar strategies were used by the administration to suppress information and dismiss or discredit scientists (Roston, 2020). With both COVID-19 and the climate crisis we see denial, delay, misinformation, and resistance to taking protective actions that would negatively impact economic growth. This pattern will continue to result in the avoidable loss of human lives.

Individualism as a shared pretense for collective inaction

Individualism is a second pretense for collective inaction shared by those who oppose collective climate action as well as those who opposed collective COVID-19 measures. Despite evidence to the contrary, it remains widely believed that if one 'does one's part' by, for example, driving a hybrid car, reducing air travel, eating vegan, using energy efficient appliances, and 'buying green,' one can stave off climate change. Addressing climate change is often said to be a matter of making lifestyle adjustments and buying green products so that individuals can influence what companies produce. As a stand-alone strategy, green consumption will not be effective at the rate and scale necessary.

Even if everyone did everything possibly to reduce individual emissions it would represent a fraction of the necessary reductions. In a widely cited study, Dietz et al. (2009) found that changes in individual and household energy use could reduce carbon emissions by more than seven percent in the US. Households are responsible for about 31% of US carbon dioxide emissions, equivalent to about 8% of global emissions (Dietz et al., 2009). Beyond reducing household energy use, individuals can adopt a range of other practices to reduce carbon emissions. Researchers estimate that a shift to 'green consumption' (choosing lower-impact products) in European countries could reduce carbon emissions by 25% (Moran et al., 2020). In a 2018 report, the Center for Behavior and the Environment estimates that the widespread adoption of 30 different behavioural changes could mitigate from 19 to 36% of global carbon emissions between 2020 and 2050 (CBE, 2018). The same report also states that about two-thirds of all global carbon emissions are linked to either direct or indirect consumption. Based on any of these estimates, the majority of global emissions remain outside of individuals' ability to influence.

It takes more than individual lifestyle changes to transform material and energy production as well as transportation infrastructure and options. For example, the reduction in global carbon emissions due to the COVID-19 pandemic lockdown was around 17% (Harvey, 2020). While some framed this reduction in a positive light, stressing that individual changes can really add up, scientists explained that 'at the same time, 83% of global emissions are left, which shows how difficult it is to reduce emissions with changes in behaviour ... Just behavioural change is not enough' (Harvey, 2020). Further, corporations, industry, and governments continue to shape individuals' options and choices pushing them to consume more and more unnecessary goods (Stuart et al., 2020b). While there are good reasons to seek out a low-carbon lifestyle (e.g. virtue ethics, increasing awareness, and demonstrating low-carbon living), a significant contribution to mitigation would require a collective commitment to many lifestyle changes. However, the danger lies in believing these efforts alone are enough to limit warming.

Especially in the US, national responses to COVID-19 also remained in line with individualism, resulting in the greatest number of cases and deaths globally (as of May 19 2021) despite being 4 percent of the world population. Without a nationally coordinated response, the Trump administration left handling the pandemic up to state governors. Some governors in conservative states either did not implement safety measures, delayed safety measures, or as in the case of states like Texas restrictions were lifted well before health officials recommended. In Texas, Governor Abbot lifted mask mandates and reopened all businesses, with health experts claiming it was far too soon (Allen & Boyette, 2021). In some states, not only were state mask mandates ended prematurely but any local mask mandates were banned.

Eichengreen (2020, p. 372) quotes an online article from the Idaho Freedom Foundation that encapsulates a widespread individualistic attitude toward the pandemic in the US: 'The decision to wear a mask should be yours alone.' It quickly became clear that if 'back to normal is up to you,' without government intervention, the pandemic would have greater impacts and last much longer. In the absence of any national policy, state-level policies were inconsistent: some states and cities imposed stay-at-home restrictions and mandates to wear masks, while others did not.

Bazzi et al. (2020) demonstrate that county-level variation is partially explained by duration of experience with the frontier conditions (total frontier experience) (TFE). Longer TFE is associated with lower rates of face mask use in public and weaker local government responses (e.g. emergency declarations and stay-at-home orders). TFE is associated with 'rugged individualism,' a combination of individualism and anti-government interventionism.

Focusing on voluntary actions and prioritizing personal freedoms before collective well-being continues to inhibit and undermine effective solutions to social and ecological crises. For many people, especially in the US, neoliberal ideology continues to make government efforts to protect citizens seem like unwanted interference and an infringement on individual rights (Harvey, 2005). The dual crises we currently face cannot be effectively addressed without large-scale coordinated actions. Klein (2014) argues that the need to address the climate crisis emerged at the worst possible historic moment: a time dominated by neoliberal ideology. However, the inability to address these crises is more than a matter of bad timing. We would likely have more protective measures in place without neoliberalism, yet the economic growth imperative would still undermine the most effective and just paths forward.

Techno-optimism as a shared pretense for collective inaction

Techno-optimism is a third pretense for collective inaction common in climate politics and pandemic responses. By techno-optimism we mean a belief or faith in technological development will solve all or most serious environmental and public health threats, even without social changes. In the cases of climate change and the COVID-19 pandemic, the widespread faith that a techno-fix can allow us to maintain the status quo and the economic growth imperative has hindered social changes that could reduce harm.

An August 2020 piece in *The Washington Post* explained that due to the dual threats of climate change and COVID-19, more people are looking to colonize Mars (Tharoor, 2020). In other words, as the Earth becomes increasingly unlivable, we should use technology to find a way out. While colonizing Mars may be an extreme example, it is rooted in a more widespread belief that technological breakthroughs will solve problems, silver bullets that eliminate the need for social change (Foster et al., 2010; Gunderson et al., 2019). Technological solutions are central to climate change mitigation strategies. One prominent form of techno-optimism in climate politics is focusing on alternative energy sources and improvements in efficiency to address climate change. What this focus fails to recognize is that improvements in efficiency tend to result in increased energy consumption and in many cases the partial or full negation of energy savings (see York & McGee, 2016). In addition, most discussions about 100% renewable energy fail to acknowledge differences in the energy return on energy invested, making it very unlikely that renewables can support current levels of energy consumption (Hall et al., 2014). Even with new technologies, effectively limiting warming requires reducing total energy consumption. Technologies will certainly be essential to minimize the impacts of climate change, yet their potential remains constrained by increasing levels of production and consumption.

A second common form of techno-optimism is much riskier. More attention, funding, and resources are being devoted to developing both solar and carbon geoengineering strategies. The most popular solar geoengineering strategy, sulfuric aerosol injection, is touted as cheap and easy but research shows it could result in drought, famine, war, and rapid warming if aerosol deposition is ever terminated (e.g. Ferraro et al., 2014; Robock, 2008; Weisenstein et al., 2015). Carbon geoengineering approaches involve removing carbon dioxide from the atmosphere, yet expectations are far ahead of actual developments. Reliance on geoengineering approaches remains risky and unreliable, yet they are increasingly included in climate models and are also supported by the fossil fuel industry, conservative politicians, and corporations (Gunderson et al., 2019 Hamilton, 2014;). It is possible that solar and carbon geoengineering will be employed in the future, as mitigation efforts remain weak and vested interests would substantially benefit from keeping the production-consumption engine accelerating. These vested interests prefer solutions that allow for economic growth and even the further extraction and use of fossil fuels (Hamilton, 2014; Kruger, 2017). The 'Promethean' proponents if geoengineering, for example, 'are inclined to see it [climate engineering] as a way of defending the established order so that expansion can continue uninterrupted' (Hamilton, 2013, p. 208). In addition, some firms hope their patented geoengineering technologies will bring in vast profits.

In the case of COVID-19, there was a similar emphasis on finding a techno-fix to the problem: the race to find a vaccine, or as Trump explained, 'protect our people from the horrible China virus' (Trump Whitehouse Archives, 2020b). Obviously, developing a vaccine is a much more viable 'silver bullet' than any technological climate change mitigation strategy. There is a stark dissimilarity between 'waiting for a vaccine' and 'waiting for 'clean coal' through carbon capture and storage,' for example, different in terms of feasibility, effectiveness, and wait-time. However, the emphasis on vaccines over social changes is still instructive as it was not only pursued to save lives but to also justify inaction and ramping up the production-consumption engine. 'Operation Warp Speed' in the US involved giving billions of dollars to biotech firms to fund accelerated vaccine development and trials. Trump's private-sector approach resulted in competition between state and federal governments and higher costs. Firms like Moderna have seen their stocks soar and are poised to make billions through intellectual property rights for their vaccine. Initial efforts to distribute the vaccine were delayed due to inconsistent state action and insufficient staff to administer them (Robbins et al., 2020). The profit motive and patents, particularly in the context of global trade agreements and developing countries, create bottlenecks and could lead to insufficient distribution this year and beyond (Labonte & Johri, 2020). Given these problems, some health experts are calling for a ban on patents, especially international patents governed by the World Trade Organization (Doucleff, 2021).

Another dimension of techno-optimism revealed prior to vaccine launches, is the longing for a silver bullet to avoid social changes and economic downturn. In the US, former President Trump pitched a number of fixes to address COVID-19, including bleach, sunlight, convalescent plasma treatment, and taking anti-malaria medication. For example, when asked if anti-malaria drug hydroxychloroquine is effect, President Trump responded: 'Many doctors think it is extremely successful – the hydroxychloroquine ... I happen to believe in it. I would take it' (Trump Whitehouse Archives, 2020b). However, the science did not support this belief (Marchione, 2020). These 'fixes' were also touted on social-media further misleading the public. The search for a quick-fix was paramount to Trump's re-election campaign, as 'promising' solutions continued to be proposed and subsequently debunked.

More importantly, even an effective solution to this particular pandemic fails to address the threat of future pandemics. For many infectious disease experts, the COVID-19 pandemic was not a surprise. Health experts have been warning for decades that a pandemic was highly likely to occur and more disease outbreaks will occur as humans increasingly transform the biosphere. Many also believe that much more severe pandemics will follow COVID-19, especially as climate change reshapes biophysical relationships and increases disease transmission, and the intensification of animal agriculture increases the likelihood of zoonoses (Humane Society International,

2020). Therefore, even an effective vaccine to *this* pandemic, is unlikely to be a long-term solution. Experts state that to avoid future pandemics we need to stop dramatically altering the climate and other biophysical relationships. As Pazaitis et al. (2020, p. 619) put it: 'Most probably the current threat will soon abate, while effective treatment and vaccines will soon be available. However, we should not feel complacent and refrain from considering the embedded problems that made our societies vulnerable in the first place.'

Faith in techno-fixes represents an ongoing pretense for collective inaction – specifically a denial that bigger social changes are necessary. Given that these techno-fixes are unlikely to offer long-term, safe, or reliable solutions (and serve to benefit the wealthy *few*), larger social changes need to be considered – social changes that could significantly improve quality of life and well-being for *all*.

Conclusion: the need for a new system

The economic growth imperative not only drives climate change and created the conditions for the development and spread of the COVID-19 pandemic but is also the context for climate change inaction and ineffective responses to the pandemic. Pretenses for collective inaction on COVID-19 are similar in content to justifications for delay in climate action: (1) denialism, (2) individualism, and (3) techno-optimism. These justifications for inaction are used to protect the same vested interests who benefit most from maintaining the economic growth imperative at the expense of the global majority. These pretenses must be widely identified as strategies to maintain the status quo and refuted. Adequately addressing climate change and future pandemics requires transitioning to social conditions that are resilient, healthy, and sustainable – leaving behind economic growth as a priority.

The growth imperative is an often-unquestioned goal of policy, as ever-increasing levels of production and consumption are necessary to accumulate capital and keep GDP increasing. Yet as prioritizing growth hinders us from effectively addressing both climate change and a global pandemic, it is time to confront these priorities. Examining the negative ecological and social costs of growth requires rethinking the structural conditions of capitalist societies (Antonio, 2009; Foster, 2011; Spash, 2020a).

The COVID-19 pandemic presents an opportunity to transition to a more sustainable society, or at least envision what a more sustainable society would look like in practice (Cohen, 2020; Rosenbloom & Markard, 2020; Sarkis et al., 2020; Yun, 2020). Even some of the behavioural changes adopted during the crisis, such as the increase in virtual meetings and conferences, should become long-term sustainability strategies (Sarkis et al., 2020). The pressing question is how to install a 'post-Covid "green recovery"' (Gills & Morgan, 2020, p. 11) that can reduce emissions while increasing well-being without relying on economic growth, and is more resistant to shocks. What would a 'Green New Deal without growth' look like (Mastini et al., 2021)? In order to prioritize life and well-being, we need structural change. This means changes that go beyond modest reforms or simple tweaks to markets and prices. It means redesigning how our economy and society function to ensure more positive outcomes. For example, a Dutch manifesto signed by 170 academics prioritizes five policy strategies to accomplish these goals:

1. 'a move away from "development" focused on aggregate GDP growth';
2. 'an economic framework focused on redistribution';
3. 'transformation towards regenerative agriculture';
4. 'reduction of consumption and travel';
5. 'debt cancellation.' (Feola, 2020)

The dual crises of climate change and the COVID-19 pandemic increasingly reveal the absurdity and immorality of our current system. Yet, Gareth Dale (2020) rightly points out that '[t]he perils of COVID-19 are trivial in comparison with those of climate breakdown and biodiversity loss.' While they share the same root driver – profit-driven transformation of the environment – the losses and suffering associated with climate change will be much greater and will also trigger new waves of novel diseases and pandemics. A widely circulated cartoon on social media illustrated this comparison through a depiction of three waves crashing upon humanity: a small wave labelled COVID-19, a second larger wave following it labelled climate change, and an even larger wave behind them both (dwarfing the others) labelled biodiversity collapse. COVID-19 has exposed important realities and trade-offs that will apply to mitigating the climate and biodiversity crises: delay only causes more harm, lack of national or global scale governance responses will cost lives, and (as illustrated clearly through the US) when leaders prioritize economic growth much more lives are unnecessarily lost. If world leaders *were* to learn from the pandemic, they would act quickly to curb carbon emissions and habitat destruction, create national and globally coordinated policies, and replace the outdated and misguided prioritization of GDP growth with the prioritization of well-being.

However, as Dale (2020) explains, both the pandemic and the climate crisis 'illustrate a troubling tendency to the downplaying of dangers where their amelioration would rub against corporate interests.' Current power relations inhibit us from most effectively and justly addressing these crises and must be confronted. It is far past time to create a new economy where people and well-being matter (Spash, 2020b). It is critical that false pretenses are identified and refuted, opening up opportunities to demand this transformation and create the social conditions to most effectively and justly address global crises.

Disclosure statement

No potential conflict of interest was reported by the author(s).

ORCID

Diana Stuart http://orcid.org/0000-0003-1479-2208
Brian Petersen http://orcid.org/0000-0003-4208-441X
Ryan Gunderson http://orcid.org/0000-0002-3837-0723

References

Agius, C., Rosamond, A. B., & Kinnvall, C. (2020). Populism, ontological insecurity and gendered nationalism: Masculinity, climate denial and Covid-19. *Politics, Religion & Ideology*, *21*(4), 432–450. https://doi.org/10.1080/21567689.2020.1851871

Allen, K., & Boyette, C. (2021, March 10). As Texas governor lifts state mask mandate, here's what we know. *CNN News*. www.cnn.com/2021/03/10/us/texas-mask-order-what-we-know/index.html

Antonio, R. J. (2009). Climate change, the resource crunch, and the global growth imperative. *Current Perspectives in Social Theory*, *26*, 3–73. https://doi.org/10.1108/S0278-1204(2009)0000026004

Antonio, R. J. (2013). Plundering the commons: The growth imperative in neoliberal times. *The Sociological Review*, *61*(2_suppl), 18–42. https://doi.org/10.1111/1467-954X.12098

Bazzi, S., Fiszbein, M., & Gebresilasse, M. (2020). *Rugged individualism and collective (in) action during the COVID-19 pandemic* (No. w27776). National Bureau of Economic Research.

Bergengruen, V., & Hennigan, W. J. (2020, October 6). You're gonna beat it.' How Donald Trump's COVID-19 battle has only fueled misinformation. *Time Magazine*. https://time.com/5896709/trump-covid-campaign/

Bhattacharya, T., & Dale, G. (2020). Covid capitalism: General tendencies, possible 'leaps'. *Spectre Journal*, *23*. https://spectrejournal.com/covid-capitalism/

Blackwater, B. (2015). Rediscovering Rosa Luxemburg. *Renewal*.

Blühdorn, I. (2007). Sustaining the unsustainable: Symbolic politics and the politics of simulation. *Environmental Politics*, *16*(2), 251–275. https://doi.org/10.1080/09644010701211759

Brulle, R. J., & Norgaard, K. M. (2019). Avoiding cultural trauma: Climate change and social inertia. *Environmental Politics*, *28*(5), 886–908. https://doi.org/10.1080/09644016.2018.1562138

Burgis, B. (2020). The left can't just dismiss the lockdown protests. *Jacobin*. https://jacobinmag.com/2020/04/coronavirus-pandemic-lockdown-protests-ubi/

Capano, G., Howlett, M., Jarvis, D. S., Ramesh, M., & Goyal, N. (2020). Mobilizing policy (in)capacity to fight COVID-19: Understanding variations in state responses. *Policy and Society*, *39*(3), 285–308. https://doi.org/10.1080/14494035.2020.1787628

Carr, P. R. (2020). If everything has changed, why such a focus on bailing out capitalism? The somber reality underpinning Covid-19. *Postdigital Science and Education*, *2*(3), 569–575. https://doi.org/10.1007/s42438-020-00115-6

Center for Behavior and the Environment. (2018). *Climate change needs behavior change*. https://www.rare.org/wp-content/uploads/2019/02/2018-CCNBC-Report.pdf

Circle Economy. (2020). https://www.circularity-gap.world/2020

Clark, B., Auerbach, D., & Longo, S. (2018). The bottom line: Capital's production of social inequalities and environmental degradation. *Journal of Environmental Studies and Sciences*, *8*, 562–569. https://doi.org/10.1007/s13412-018-0505-6

Cohen, M. J. (2020). Does the COVID-19 outbreak mark the onset of a sustainable consumption transition? *Sustainability*, *16*, 1–3. https://doi.org/10.1080/15487733.2020.1740472

Dale, G. (2020). Karl Polanyi, the new deal, and the green new deal. *Environmental Values*. Advance online publication. https://doi.org/10.3197/096327120X16033868459485

Daly, H. (1973). *Toward a steady-state economy*. Freeman.

Dietz, T. (2015). Prolegomenon to a structural human ecology of human well-being. *Sociology of Development*, *1*(1), 123–148. https://doi.org/10.1525/sod.2015.1.1.123

Dietz, T., Gardner, G. T., Gilligan, J., Stern, P. C., & Vandenbergh, M. P. (2009). Household actions can provide a behavioral wedge to rapidly reduce US carbon emissions. *Proceedings of the National Academy of Sciences*, *106*(44), 18452–18456. https://doi.org/10.1073/pnas.0908738106

Doucleff, M. (2021). What will it take to end the COVID-19 pandemic? NPR. https://www.npr.org/sections/goatsandsoda/2021/01/05/953653373/some-experts-say-temporary-halt-on-drug-patents-is-needed-to-stop-pandemic-world

Dunlap, R. E., & Brulle, R. J. (Eds.). (2015). *Climate change and society: Sociological perspectives*. Oxford University Press.

Dunlap, R. E., McCright, A. M., & Yarosh, J. H. (2016). The political divide on climate change: Partisan polarization widens in the US. *Environment: Science and Policy for Sustainable Development*, *58*(5), 4–23. https://doi.org/10.1080/00139157.2016.1208995

Eichengreen, B. (2020). Individualism, polarization and recovery from the COVID-19 crisis. *Intereconomics*, 55(6), 371–374. https://doi.org/10.1007/s10272-020-0928-7

Falkenbach, M., & Greer, S. L. (2020). Denial and distraction: How the populist radical right responds to COVID-19; comment on "a scoping review of PRR parties' influence on welfare policy and its implication for population health in Europe". *International Journal of Health Policy and Management*, https://doi.org/10.34172/ijhpm.2020.141

Feola, G. (2020). Manifesto for post-neoliberal development: Five policy strategies for the Netherlands after the Covid-19 crisis. Ontgroei. https://ontgroei.degrowth.net/manifesto-for-post-neoliberal-development-five-policy-strategies-for-the-netherlands-after-the-covid-19-crisis/

Ferraro, A. J., Highwood, E. J., & Charlton-Perez, A. J. (2014). Weakened tropical circulation and reduced precipitation in response to geoengineering. *Environmental Research Letters*, 9(1), 014001. https://doi.org/10.1088/1748-9326/9/1/014001

Foster, J. B. (2011). Capitalism and degrowth: An impossibility theorem. *Monthly Review*, 62(8), 26–33. https://doi.org/10.14452/MR-062-08-2011-01_2

Foster, J. B., Clark, B., & York, R. (2010). *The ecological rift: Capitalism's war on the earth*. Monthly Review Press.

Fuentes, R., Galeotti, M., Lanza, A., & Manzano, B. (2020). COVID-19 and climate change: A tale of two global problems. *Sustainability*, 12(20), 8560. https://doi.org/10.3390/su12208560

Georgescu-Roegen, N. (1971). *The entropy law and the economic process*. Harvard University Press.

Giddens, A. (2009). *Politics of climate change*. Polity.

Gills, B., & Morgan, J. (2020). Economics and climate emergency. *Globalizations*. Advance online publication. https://doi.org/10.1080/14747731.2020.1841527

Gunderson, R., Stuart, D., & Petersen, B. (2019). The political economy of geoengineering as plan B: Technological rationality, moral hazard, and new technology. *New Political Economy*, 24(5), 696–715. https://doi.org/10.1080/13563467.2018.1501356

Hall, C. A., Lambert, J. G., & Balogh, S. B. (2014). EROI of different fuels and the implications for society. *Energy Policy*, 64, 141–152. https://doi.org/10.1016/j.enpol.2013.05.049

Hamilton, C. (2004). *Growth fetish*. Pluto Press.

Hamilton, C. (2013). *Earthmasters: The dawn of the age of climate engineering*. Yale University Press.

Hamilton, C. (2014). Geoengineering and the politics of science. *Bulletin of the Atomic Scientists*, 70(3), 17–26. https://doi.org/10.1177/0096340214531173

Harvey, D. (2005). *A brief history of neoliberalism*. Oxford University Press.

Harvey, F. (2020, May 19). Lockdown triggers dramatic fall in global carbon emissions. *The Guardian*. https://www.theguardian.com/environment/2020/may/19/lockdowns-trigger-dramatic-fall-global-carbon-emissions

Hauck, G. (2020, September 18). CDC now recommends all people exposed to COVID-19 get tested, reversing earlier controversial guidance. *USA Today*. https://www.usatoday.com/story/news/health/2020/09/18/covid-testing-cdc-reverses-guidelines-asymptomatic-spread/5827365002/

Henley, J. (2020, November 12). Swedish surge in Covid cases dashes immunity hopes. *The Guardian*. https://www.theguardian.com/world/2020/nov/12/covid-infections-in-sweden-surge-dashing-hopes-of-herd-immunity

Hickel, J. (2017). *The divide: A brief guide to global inequality and its solutions*. Random House.

Hickel, J., & Kallis, G. (2020). Is Green growth possible? *New Political Economy*, 25(4), 469–486. https://doi.org/10.1080/13563467.2019.1598964

Horta-Barba, A., Kulisevsky, J., & Marín-Lahoz, J. (2020). Is COVID-19 expansion a consequence of a group inaction. *J Med Public Health*, 1(1), 1006.

Humane Society International. (2020). The connection between animal agriculture, viral zoonoses, and global pandemics. https://www.hsi.org/wp-content/uploads/2020/10/Animal-agriculture-viral-disease-and-pandemics.pdf

IPCC. (2018). Summary for policymakers. In V. Masson-Delmotte, P. Zhai, H.-O. Pörtner, D. Roberts, J. Skea, P. R. Shukla, A. Pirani, W. Moufouma-Okia, C. Péan, R. Pidcock, S. Connors, J. B. R. Matthews, Y. Chen, X. Zhou, M. I. Gomis, E. Lonnoy, T. Maycock, M. Tignor, and T. Waterfield (Eds.), *Global warming of 1.5°C. An IPCC special report on the impacts of global warming of 1.5°C above pre-industrial levels and related global greenhouse gas emission pathways, in the context of strengthening the global response to the threat of climate change, sustainable development, and efforts to eradicate poverty* (p. 3–24). World Meteorological Organization.

John Hopkins Coronavirus Resource Center. (2021). Retrieved May 19, 2021, from https://coronavirus.jhu.edu/map.html

Klein, N. (2014). *This changes everything: Capitalism vs. the climate.* Simon and Schuster.

Koch, M., & Buch-Hansen, H. (2020). In search of a political economy of the postgrowth era. *Globalizations*, 1–11. https://doi.org/10.1080/14747731.2020.1807837

Kruger, T. (2017). Conflicts over carbon capture and storage in international climate governance. *Energy Policy*, *100*, 58–67. https://doi.org/10.1016/j.enpol.2016.09.059

Labonte, R., & Johri, M. (2020). COVID-19 drug and vaccine patents are putting profit before people. *The Conversation*. Retrieved January 26, 2021, from https://theconversation.com/covid-19-drug-and-vaccine-patents-are-putting-profit-before-people-149270

Mann, M. E. (2021). *The new climate war: The fight to take back the planet.* Public Affairs.

Manzanedo, R. D., & Manning, P. (2020). COVID-19: Lessons for the climate change emergency. *Science of the Total Environment*, *742*, 140563. https://doi.org/10.1016/j.scitotenv.2020.140563

Marchione, M. (2020, June 3). Malaria drug fails to prevent COVID-19 in a rigorous study. *AP News*. https://apnews.com/article/malaria-donald-trump-us-news-ap-top-news-virus-outbreak-acdfd2d1fda245315a164225d15d360c

Markard, J., & Rosenbloom, D. (2020). A tale of two crises: COVID-19 and climate. *Sustainability: Science, Practice and Policy*, *16*(1), 53–60. https://doi.org/10.1080/15487733.2020.1765679

Mastini, R., Kallis, G., & Hickel, J. (2021). A green new deal without growth? *Ecological Economics*, *179*, 106832. https://doi.org/10.1016/j.ecolecon.2020.106832

Meeker, J. K. (2020). *The ironic resistance of anti-quarantine protesters. COVID-19: Volume II: Social consequences and cultural adaptations.* Routledge.

Miller, B. L. (2020). Science denial and COVID conspiracy theories: Potential neurological mechanisms and possible responses. *JAMA*, *324*(22), 2255–2256. https://doi.org/10.1001/jama.2020.21332

Modonesi, C. (2020). The environmental roots of zoonotic diseases: From SARS-CoV-2 to cancer viruses. A review. *Visions for Sustainability*, *14*, 54–65. https://doi.org/10.13135/2384-8677/5319

Moran, D., Wood, R., Hertwich, E., Mattson, K., Rodriguez, J. F., Schanes, K., & Barrett, J. (2020). Quantifying the potential for consumer-oriented policy to reduce European and foreign carbon emissions. *Climate Policy*, 20(Sup 1), S28–S38. https://doi.org/10.1080/14693062.2018.1551186

Newell, R., & Dale, A. (2020). COVID-19 and climate change: An integrated perspective. *Cities & Health*, https://doi.org/10.1080/23748834.2020.1778844

Ollinaho, O. I. (2016). Environmental destruction as (objectively) uneventful and (subjectively) irrelevant. *Environmental Sociology*, *2*(1), 53–63. https://doi.org/10.1080/23251042.2015.1114207

Ott, C. K. (2018). On the political economy of solar radiation management. *Frontiers in Environmental Science*, 1–13. https://doi.org/10.3389/fenvs.2018.00043

Oxfam. (2018). https://www.oxfam.org/en/press-releases/richest-1-percent-bagged-82-percent-wealth-created-last-year-poorest-half-humanity

Parrique, T., Barth, J., Briens, F., Kerschner, C., Kraus-Polk, A., Kuokkanen, A., & Spangenberg, J. H. (2019). Decoupling debunked: Evidence and arguments against green growth as a sole strategy for sustainability. European Environmental Bureau.

Pazaitis, A., Kostakis, V., Kallis, G., & Troullaki, K. (2020). Should we look for a hero to save us from the coronavirus? The commons as an alternative trajectory for social change. *tripleC*, *18*(2), 613–621. https://doi.org/10.31269/triplec.v18i2.1203

Petersen, B., Stuart, D., & Gunderson, R. (2019). Reconceptualizing climate change denial: Ideological denialism misdiagnoses climate change and limits effective action. *Human Ecology Review*, *25*(2), 117–141. https://doi.org/10.22459/HER.25.02.2019.08

Popovich, N., Albeck-Ripka, L. and Pierre-Louis, K. (2021, January 20). The Trump administration rolled back more than 100 environmental rules. Here's the full list. *New York Times*. https://www.nytimes.com/interactive/2020/climate/trump-environment-rollbacks-list.html

Ripple, W. J., Wolf, C., Newsome, T. M., Barnard, P., & Moomaw, W. R. (2020). World scientists' warning of a climate emergency. *BioScience*, *70*(1), 8–12. https://academic.oup.com/bioscience/article/70/1/8/5610806?searchresult=1

Robbins, R., Robles, F., & Arango, T. (2020, December 31). Here's why distribution of the vaccine is taking longer than expected. *The New York Times*.

Robertson, R. (2020). Humanity for itself? Reflections on climate change and the Covid-19 pandemic. *Globalizations*, 1–9. https://doi.org/10.1080/14747731.2020.1842684

Robock, A. (2008). 20 reasons why geoengineering may be a bad idea. *Bulletin of the Atomic Scientists*, *64*(2), 14–59. https://doi.org/10.1080/00963402.2008.11461140

Rocco, P., Béland, D., & Waddan, A. (2020). Stuck in neutral? Federalism, policy instruments, and counter-cyclical responses to COVID-19 in the United States. *Policy and Society*, *39*(3), 458–477. https://doi.org/10.1080/14494035.2020.1783793

Rosenbloom, D., & Markard, J. (2020). A COVID-19 recovery for climate. *Science*, *368*(6490), 447. https://doi.org/10.1126/science.abc4887

Roston, E. (2020, July 20). Science is collateral damage across the Trump administration. *Bloomberg News*. https://www.bloomberg.com/news/articles/2020-07-20/science-is-collateral-damage-across-the-trump-administration

Ruiu, M. L., Ragnedda, M., & Ruiu, G. (2020). Similarities and differences in managing the Covid-19 crisis and climate change risk. *Journal of Knowledge Management*, *24*(10), 2597–2614. https://doi.org/10.1108/JKM-06-2020-0492

Sarkis, J., Cohen, M. J., Dewick, P., & Schröder, P. (2020). A brave new world: Lessons from the COVID-19 pandemic for transitioning to sustainable supply and production. *Resources, Conservation and Recycling*, *159*, 104894. https://doi.org/10.1016/j.resconrec.2020.104894

Schnaiberg, A. (1980). *The environment: From surplus to scarcity*. Oxford University Press.

Schor, J. B., & Jorgenson, A. K. (2019). Is it too late for growth? *Review of Radical Political Economics*, *51*(2), 320–329. https://doi.org/10.1177/0486613419831109

Semuels, A. (2016, November 4). Does the economy really need to keep growing quite so much? *The Atlantic*. https://www.theatlantic.com/business/archive/2016/11/economic-growth/506423/

Shannon, J. (2020, April 3). Americans support drastic efforts to stop coronavirus, expect crisis to last for months in Public Agenda/USA TODAY/Ipsos poll. *USA Today*. https://www.usatoday.com/in-depth/news/nation/2020/04/03/coronavirus-poll-americans-saving-lives-economy-public-agenda/5098766002/

Spash, C. L. (2020a). Apologists for growth: Passive revolutionaries in a passive revolution. *Globalizations*. Advance online publication. https://doi.org/10.1080/14747731.2020.1824864

Spash, C. L. (2020b). 'The economy' as if people mattered: Revisiting critiques of economic growth in a time of crisis. *Globalizations*. Advance online publication. https://doi.org/10.1080/14747731.2020.1761612

Speth, J. G. (2008). *The bridge at the end of the world: Capitalism, the environment, and crossing from crisis to sustainability*. Yale University Press.

Steffen, W., Rockström, J., Richardson, K., Lenton, T. M., Folke, C., Liverman, D., Summerhayes, C. P., Barnosky, A. D., Cornell, S. E., Crucifix, M., Donges, J. F., Fetzer, I., Lade, S. J., Scheffer, M., Winkelmann, R., & Schellnhuber, H. J. (2018). Trajectories of the earth system in the anthropocene. *Proceedings of the National Academy of Sciences*, *115*(33), 8252–8259. https://doi.org/10.1073/pnas.1810141115

Stern, P. C., Perkins, J. H., Sparks, R. E., & Knox, R. A. (2016). The challenge of climate-change neoskepticism. *Science*, *353*(6300), 653–654. https://doi.org/10.1126/science.aaf6675

Stiglitz, J. E. (2009, September 12). The great GDP swindle. *The Guardian*. https://www.theguardian.com/commentisfree/2009/sep/13/economics-economic-growth-and-recession-global-economy

Stiglitz, J. E. (2019, November 24). It's time to retire metrics like GDP. They don't measure everything that matters. *The Guardian*. https://www.theguardian.com/commentisfree/2019/nov/24/metrics-gdp-economic-performance-social-progress

Stoner, A. M., & Melathopoulos, A. (2015). *Freedom in the anthropocene: Twentieth-century helplessness in the face of climate change*. Palgrave Macmillan.

Stuart, D., Gunderson, R., & Petersen, B. (2020a). *The degrowth alternative: A path to address our environmental crisis?* Routledge.

Stuart, D., Gunderson, R., & Petersen, B. (2020b). Overconsumption as ideology: Implications for addressing global climate change. *Nature and Culture*, *15*(2), 199–223. https://doi.org/10.3167/nc.2020.150205

Tharoor, I. (2020, July 28). As crises rock earth, humans look to mars. *The Washington Post*. https://www.washingtonpost.com/world/2020/07/29/crises-rock-earth-humans-look-mars/

Trump White House Archives. (2017, June 1). Statement by President Trump on the Paris climate accord. https://trumpwhitehouse.archives.gov/briefings-statements/statement-president-trump-paris-climate-accord/

Trump White House Archives. (2020a, November 13). Remarks by President Trump during an update on operation warp speed, https://trumpwhitehouse.archives.gov/briefings-statements/remarks-president-trump-update-operation-warp-speed/

Trump White House Archives. (2020b, July 28). Remarks by President Trump in press briefing, https://trumpwhitehouse.archives.gov/briefings-statements/remarks-president-trump-press-briefing-july-28-2020/

Urry, J. (2011). *Climate change & society*. Polity.

Weisenstein, D. K., Keith, D. W., & Dykema, J. A. (2015). Solar geoengineering using solid aerosol in the stratosphere. *Atmospheric Chemistry and Physics*, *15*(20), 11835–11859. https://doi.org/10.5194/acp-15-11835-2015

Worland, J. (2017, April 12). Climate change deniers have President Trump's ear. But now they want results. *Time Magazine*. https://time.com/4712153/climate-change-deniers-donald-trump-epa-global-warming/

Wright, E. O. (2010). *Envisioning real utopias* (Vol. 98). Verso.

York, R., & McGee, J. A. (2016). Understanding the jevons paradox. *Environmental Sociology*, *2*(1), 77–87. https://doi.org/10.1080/23251042.2015.1106060

Yun, S.-J. (2020, October 16). *Lessons of COVID-10: Toward metamorphosis to deal with climate change* [Paper presentation]. 2020 Pusan National University Graduate School of Climate Change International Conference, Busan, South Korea.

On living in an already-unsettled world: COVID as an expression of larger transformations

Paul James ⓘ and Manfred B. Steger ⓘ

ABSTRACT
This essay elaborates the terms of our central argument about the current intensification of global disjunctures. We introduce a crucial dimension of our engaged theory of globalization that can usefully be brought to the fore to understand these cleavages and tensions. The essay scrutinizes two key conjunctures, comparing the current Global Covid Crisis with the 2008–2009 Global Financial Crisis. It concludes that massive disjunctures in the way we live locally and globally have had incongruous effects on the global-local nexus, but without leading to positive transformation. Rather, they are both expressions of a longer-term transformation we have been calling the Great Unsettling. Without reflexive counter-practices, the most likely mid-term prognosis for the world is an intensification of tensions and disjunctures that are leading to a further thickening of this complex dynamic.

It is tempting to see the current COVID-19 pandemic as curtailing global capitalism, or at least challenging unsustainable long-distance trade networks and offshore production. Given the health risks of globalizing commodity-handling systems, surely established transnational trade practices will be deprioritized in favour of re-creating regional and local exchanges (Livesay, 2017). In light of this unprecedented health crisis, surely neoliberalism will sooner or later be caught up in its own contradictions as it continues to administer Keynesian therapy in the form of disaster welfarism combined with massive corporate bailouts. After all, these policy directions are, in theory at least, ideologically anathema to the neoliberal precepts of deregulated, efficient markets and the minimal state. Moreover, have not the current dialectics of history given people a taste of possible alternatives that had been previously relegated to the misty regions of socialist utopias abounding with steady employment support programmes and universal basic income schemes? As a result, might not citizens in the 2020s be more open to new redistributive regimes that respond even more vigorously to the growing inequalities plaguing the local-global nexus?

For an unprecedented moment, the Global Covid Crisis (GCC) also seems to have prefigured a transitional pathway to a more ecologically sustainable world. This trajectory appears to have been turbocharged with the 2020 United States electoral victory of Joe Biden. The health calamity's unintended short-term consequences – less cars on the road, less industrial output, less coal-use, less pollution in the atmosphere, and declining carbon-emissions – seem to offer a glimpse of what the global justice movement has long promised: another world is possible. This ecological scenario has been reinforced by amazing stories of elephants ambling through a village in Yunnan, China, and sea-life returning to the waters of the previously tourist-infested coastlines of the Italian Adriatic. For a few months, we witnessed the radically diminished levels of nitrogen dioxide, air particulates, water pollution, and carbon emissions in the world's major cities.

Unfortunately, however, the long-term future is uncertain. Most of the early stories of environmental hope were a bit fanciful and at times quite exaggerated. For example, the swans frequenting the famous Burano canals of the Venetian lagoon were regulars, and the footage of frolicking dolphins was not filmed in Venice, but rather at a pristine inlet on the island of Sardinia more than 700 kilometres away.

The wave of hope surging especially through global cyberspace perhaps indicates more about people's desire for positive signs than probable long-term changes. It is equally possible, for example, that the global decline in pollutants is no more than a reprise of the period of the 2008–2009 Global Financial Crisis (GFC) when parallel changes in pollution and carbon emissions registered briefly before rebounding to higher levels during the 'recovery' years (Mandal et al., 2020; Peters et al., 2012). Indeed, CNN and other global news outlets have referred to this phenomenon as 'revenge pollution' (Wright, 2020). While we do not wish to deflate the soaring spirits of those who focus on signs of hope, it seems prudent to heed Antonio Gramsci's counsel of tempering of the 'optimism of the will' with the 'pessimism of the intellect' (1971, p. 175).

What we can say with tempered confidence is that the COVID-19 pandemic has shocked the global system, and long-term positive change will depend, as always, on integrated and reflexive ecological, economic, political, and cultural action. Positive transformation will rely on collective responses in the face of the intensifying unsettling of the global-local nexus. Placed within the possible context of alternative politics, hope returns as a transitional practice directed towards alternative kinds of social engagement. In these terms, the Global Covid Crisis is not in itself enough to shock us to turn to viable alternative, certainly not in structural terms. Rather than embracing naïve hope or falling into premature despair, the point is to set up the conditions for a better world. The pandemic has unevenly intensified the enduring tensions and disjunctures of our contemporary globalized world. These disjunctures – which we will discuss in a moment – run so deep that an alternative politics that does not take them into account will quickly lose ground (Steger & James, 2020). Even political movements that experience immediate success – as diverse as Alter-Globalization, the Arab Spring, the Occupy Movement, Extinction Rebellion, and Black Lives Matter – will struggle to reverse long-term trajectories of exploitation, inequality and ecological degradation.

Accordingly, the first part of this essay elaborates the terms of our argument about the current intensification of global disjunctures. We introduce a dimension of our engaged theory of globalization that can usefully be brought to the fore to understand these cleavages and tensions (Steger & James, 2019). The essay then goes on to draw comparisons and parallels between the current Global Covid Crisis and the Global Financial Crisis. This comparison allows to show that both crises are part of a bigger existential shift in the human and planetary condition.

Intensifying global tensions and disjunctures

In our previous work, we introduced the concept of the 'Great Unsettling' – shorthand for the complex social dynamics of instability and volatility (Steger & James, 2019, 2020). This shift is far more embracing than for example Karl Polanyi's (1944) institutionally based analysis of what he called the 'Great Transformation', the collapse of four European institutions: the international gold standard, the self-regulating market, the balance-of-power system, and the liberal state. The Great Unsettling is a global dynamic that includes yet goes beyond such limited institutionally framed political economic changes. Taken together and understood in terms of the human condition, we argue that we face massive destabilization based on the ontological reconstitution of the basic conditions of living on this planet. This unsettling is described in a moment using quite conventional categories – ecologically, economically, politically and culturally – but that is just to use a familiar way into narrative. The key point in each of these descriptive domain-related accounts is that the unsettling transcends both those categories and their short-term crises to involve disjunctures in the ontological bases of life.

Ecologically, it is not just that we are pumping carbon into the atmosphere, but also that technoscientific interventions are taking apart and re-combining the basic elements of nature. This is setting up an ontological disjuncture between nature as given (including human bodies as part of nature) and nature as reconstituted by human intervention. Even the concept of 'the Anthropocene' as presently conceived does not address this process. Whether setting up conditions for hyper-exploitation of the planet *or* deploying synthetic biology and climate engineering to save it, technoscience is now fundamentally unsettling all planetary systems (Wodak, 2020). This is signaled, and ironically reinforced, in all those writings that now talk of the 'end of nature', going back to Bill McKibben's bestseller that bears this title (1989).

Economically, instruments for abstracting value such as the esoteric derivatives that almost brought down the world economy in 2008 are not just creating inequalities of wealth, but also wrenching the basis on which classical capitalism was built. In particular, the relation between abstracted risk-management/valuing and those processes of material production and exchange continues to occur in what is now somewhat quaintly (and wrongly) distinguished as 'the *real* economy'. At times of crisis, such as the GFC, this disjuncture between the cybernetic capitalism and more embodied economic practice can be overtly seen to play out in damaging ways, but for the most part the gathering dominance of digital fiduciary capital races on.

Politically, disruptions to the meaning of political representation are not just giving succor to populists, but also confirming longer-term and profound assaults on basic understandings of good governance, political truth and state legitimacy. This means that the very techniques used to build legitimacy – from algorithmic targeting to preference sampling – are undermining the long-term legitimacy of all public and private regimes. In a parallel way, institutions such as the state that once were turned to as ensuring security now carry the genesis of our deepening domestic and international insecurity.

And *culturally*, beyond the current crises of identity, transformations of what were once relatively taken-for-granted frames of meaning and enquiry are now relativizing the meaning of social life in general. There is no doubt that the Global Covid Crisis, in particular, has further intensified both people's *subjective* sense of insecurity *and* feelings that things could be otherwise. But that is not the overriding consideration we want to emphasize here. The ontological insecurity that we point to is both longer-term and world-historical, a disjuncture between meaning as being 'there' to be found (through techniques ranging from deeper personal introspection or more precise technoscientific measurement) and meaning as becoming increasingly relative to the searcher.

The ways in which the Great Unsettling has intensified is not immediately obvious. However, the extent that commentaries remain focused on the immediate consequences of different crises rather than their social-natural fracturing, they miss a key and paradoxical point. The multiple and proliferating social crises of the last few decades – the current pandemic, the 2015–2018 European and American immigration crises, the 2007–2009 GFC and the ensuing European Sovereign Debt

Crisis, the 2000 Dotcom crisis, the 1997–1998 Asian Financial Crisis, and so on – are outcomes of larger transformations, and, in themselves, not more than proximate causes of much social disruption and pain.

In these terms, the existential significance of the Global Covid Crisis is not that it introduces a completely new threat. Rather, it reveals in an indirect manner the ways in which humans have contributed to the basic disruption of our complex ecology over a long period and how this degradation has *intensified* along the disjunctures just described. Emerging evidence now suggests that dominant ways of living on this planet – intensification of industrial-digital agriculture, destruction of habitat for wild animals, trade in exotic species, reduction of species diversity, proliferation of carbon emissions and intensifying climate change[1] – have been significantly exacerbating the possibility, frequency, and generalizing impact of viral outbreaks such as COVID-19. Even if the current health crisis is consuming most of our attention, we should remember the emergence of similar threats in the last few decades such as Ebola, Zika, MERS-CoV, H1N1, SARS, and HIV-AIDS – all coming out of the same basic disjuncture between the social and the natural, and leading to a combined death toll of tens of millions of people. This means that for all the emphasis on Chinese wet markets and zoonotic transfer as the proximate source of the COVID-19 emergence, it is the intensification of hyper-consumption, destruction of our ecology, and global hypermobility that provide a more basic explanation of the proliferation of global pandemics.

This point feeds into the first core proposition in our overall argument. If the processes of the Great Unsettling have objectively contributed to the Global Covid Crisis – and not just the other way around – then, all things being equal, we are likely on both the local and global level to see enduring and intensifying circles of social conflict and tension. As a result, the Covid crisis should be seen an adumbration of a world of *continuing* and *intensifying* disjunctures. We use 'adumbration' here in the sense of a darkening picture without clear trajectories, rather than as a harbinger that foreshadows *new* transformations. Moreover, our suggestion that the Great Unsettling is a continuing process does not mean more of the same in the sense of 'business as usual', but rather an elaboration of disjunctures that have been relatively continuous *but* intensifying over the last few decades. As always, one would expect to see the appearance of new elements, but the evidence from recent crisis trajectories, even COVID-19, suggests that these emergences will amount to little more than associated changes rather than full-scale paradigmatic transformations.

Ironically, the increasing conflict over the expressive outcomes of existential matters will probably slow down the possibilities for *positive* transformation. It is probable, for example, that across the next decade the 'need' for capitalism will be both asserted more strongly by some and contested more vigorously by others. It is possible that neoliberalism will move more discordantly between instituting short-term instances of disaster welfarism, rhetorically responding to calls for empathy, and allowing ever-harsher austerity cycles to be ushered into being by capitalist 'reality'. This austerity is less likely to be directed as enunciated policy as in the past, but will most likely come about quietly due to government prioritization, particularly the redirection of state funds to reinvigorate the market.

At the same time, as William Robinson (2020) has pointed out, this less rhetorically charged economic austerity is likely to go hand in hand with the rise of a 'global police state' that uses a variety of insidious methods of social control – 'security' that makes us more ontologically insecure. Thus, in this context of uncertainty and ambiguity, it is difficult to predict whether common populist failures to curtail the spread of COVID-19 will lose elections or carry on for a time. We know that COVID-19 was a major factor in Donald Trump's downfall, but the jury is still out on Jair Bolsonaro, Boris Johnson, Victor Órban, Andrzej Duda, and many others. What seems certain, however, is that national populists *and* liberal progressives alike will have to face an intensifying legitimation crisis of the sort first described for us by Jürgen Habermas (1988) half a century ago.

Hence, derived from our first proposition, we suggest that *positive* transformation will only occur only through the slow and uneven process of effectively responding to the layered *ontological* dimensions of the Great Unsettling. This suggestion is linked to a second proposition. Over the past decades, stretching back to the middle of the twentieth century, disembodied relations – that is, relations mediated by codes and signs including digital technology – have come to overlay and fundamentally remake more embodied and material processes of global integration and interchange. This remaking is so comprehensive as to transform the human planetary condition. Put simply, the more disembodied the relation or process has become, the more it serves as an effective means to power. Conversely, the more embodied the relation, the more it is constrained, controlled, codified, regulated, surveyed, and/or exploited by digitalized surveillance regimes.

We need to take a step back to make this part of our argument clearer. This second proposition rests on an analytic method deployed in our efforts to develop an engaged theory of globalization that distinguishes different levels of social integration/differentiation (Steger & James, 2019, 2020). Our framework begins with *embodied relations* between people, where the abiding 'presence' of others predominates as the basis of the relation. Embodied relations are overlaid by *object-extended relations*, stretched further across time and space through the mediation of things ranging from commodities to viruses. Next, *institutionally extended relations* are amplified and drawn out through the practices of the agents of institutions and organizations including empires, states, and corporations. On the most abstract end of our analytical spectrum, we identified *disembodied* relations, mediated today by digital technology that overlay embodied relations in multiple and complex ways. These kinds of relations range from capital transactions to Facebook 'friendships', which often characteristically develop between acquaintances, even strangers, at short and long distances. Bringing together finance and Facebook in this way sounds provocative, but we are working at the analytic level of dominant, emergent and continuing integrational social formations, not at a descriptive level of the complex intersections of any instance or sequence of interchange. Our method encompasses yet goes beyond Adam Arvidsson's insightful observation that 'the *modus operandi* of Facebook mirrors the operations of derivative financial instruments' (2016, p. 3). Our emphasis on social form dovetails with Marshall McLuhan's (1994) graphic evocation of 'the medium is the message': form is encompassing of content; social form frames the meaning of content and has meaning in itself.

In practice, any particular act, relation, or social process is framed by the uneven intersection of these various forms – not by a single way of relating. Historically, the first three forms – embodied, object-extended, and institutionally extended – have predominated (though it should be noted that some disembodied forms of interchange such as practices of writing and print go far back in human history [James, 2020]). For present purposes, the crux of this claim is that the much more recent phenomenon of digital interchange has in the contemporary period become the *sin qua non* of disembodied relations. Through digital interchange, disembodied relations now increasingly dominate the other three forms of relation. And this domination has set up new disjunctures, both in terms of relations and power. Facebook and the possibility for power through data-mining is just one example that shows how both algorithmically and socially, the disembodied medium devours embodied relations (while being lived by some individuals as enhancing their intimate connectivity) and fractures the relation between public and private institutions (while being proclaimed by some as the basis of a new civil dialogue).

To briefly test our two main arguments – first, that the Great Unsettling will continue to intensify through the GCC and beyond; and, second, that the long-term process through which more abstract relations have come to dominate more embodied relations will also intensify – let us compare the outcomes of a major previous crisis with the current GCC. We have selected the 2008–2009 GFC for a number of reasons. Most obviously, like the Covid pandemic, its reach and consequences were global. Just as importantly, the two crises have been chosen as apparently so different as to make our task of drawing common ground as hard as meaningfully possible. Temporally, this choice allows us to compare the present moment with another period far enough in the past to assess its the outcomes and ramifications. We can thus set base-line comparisons that make the separation of a decade useful, but without the event being too distant in history for the comparison to be stretched beyond the terms that a conjunctural and integrational analysis can meaningfully handle. Moreover, we can also move comfortably between theoretical analysis and empirical thick description, just as we can move between objective and subjective phenomena. In this respect, Yanis Varoufakis's (2011, p. 3) comment about the initial subjective 'shared aporia' in response to the GFC seems to us, for example, to also apply most acutely to the GCC:

> Thus, we entered a state of tangible, shared aporia. Anxious disbelief replaced intellectual indolence. The figures in authority seemed bereft of authority. Policy was, evidently, being made on the hoof. Almost immediately, a puzzled public trained its antennae in every possible direction, desperately seeking explanations for the causes and nature of what had just hit it.

Despite profound and important differences between the two crises, we want to argue that there are some key parallels that warrant investigation in themselves. It may be unusual to put these parallels in the way that we do, but it allows for a depth of analysis that is capable of both interlinking and moving across ecological, economic, political and cultural domains. Let us begin our comparison by focusing first on the disjuncture between embodied placement and abstracted relations, and then on the disjuncture between embodied power and mediated power.

The disjuncture between embodied placement and abstracted relations

Both the GFC and the GCC have in very broad terms, we argue, involved an intensification of local-global disjunctures between placed embodied relations and more abstracted relations of globalizing accounting. Let us begin with the GFC. Despite continuing heated debates, the basic contours and evolution of the GFC are well established. In descriptive terms, the crisis began in the United States with the gradual bursting of the housing-price bubble in 2006, leading to the 2007 subprime mortgage crisis with a sharp rise in mortgage foreclosures. It spread globally, carried by a crisis of liquidity, speculation and over-borrowing, amplified by the unregulated globalization of esoteric financial securities and derivatives such as credit default swaps and collaterized debt obligations. For all of their incredible complexity and despite differences of interpretation and emphasis, this is basically how the crisis has been described in most of the literature ranging from economists (Read, 2009), political economy critics (Nesvetailova, 2007), and historians (Tooze, 2019) to cultural anthropologists (Langley, 2015). Most of the literature in this area tends to operate in the realm of middle-range theory. However, taking the analysis *both* closer to the ground of embodied relations and more abstractly into the ethereal realm of global finance capitalism, we can discern some significant disjunctures.

From the perspective of the local – even during the heights of the GFC – each activity of buying a home in a local neighbourhood continued to be enacted, *at the level of embodied placement*, as a tangible relation of intimate home-making – though, of course, within the institutional framing of moneylenders and legal requirements. Locality remained salient. Defaulting mortgages were focused, in the first instance, in very particular American locales: Riverside, Bakersfield, Stockton, Las Vegas, Modesto, Fresno, Visalia, and Phoenix – in the West of the United States, mostly in California – and Cape Coral, Orlando, and Miami in Florida (Mayer & Pence, 2008). In other words, one element of the crisis related to particular loans afforded to particular people and focused in particular localities.

More importantly for how power operates, however, these loans were lifted out of embodied placement and linked to global sub-prime mortgage financing as part of a disembodied process that had been happening for a couple of decades and had repercussions that continued beyond the GFC. Innovative *Financial Times* journalists have tracked the financial path of one particular house, 418 Homeplace Drive in Stockbridge, Georgia, showing how it left the local loan system and passed through the global 'hands' of a banker working for *Société Générale* in Paris when that bank decided to bet on mortgage defaults. Coming back to the local embodied, Trevor and Colleen Pace, the owners of the house, finally succumbed in 2013 to the wave of foreclosures, thus joining the 7.8 million families in the United States that were dispossessed between 2007 and 2016. Trevor and Colleen have since separated, linking personal tragedy even more closely to abstract global financial flows (Vandevelde et al., 2018).

How did such a place-based and intimately embodied activity become caught up in a broader process in which the institutions of mortgage lending had become radically extended spatially and systematically abstracted from the persons and objects on the ground? From about the 1960s, large national lending institutions emerged unevenly, gradually supplanting local loan processes. Then, taking off in the 1980s, mortgages began to be bundled far beyond the local event as abstracted globalized securities (Aalbers, 2009). Residential mortgage-backed securities, or RMBS, were presented in the first instance in the 1970s by government-sponsored institutions such as Fannie Mae and Freddie Mac as a means of offsetting local risk. But let us note here that the concept of 'local' had by this time come to mean something quite different from the neighbourhoods where people buy homes. RMBS expanded rapidly in the early 2000s for a very different reason: making money. In the 2000s, new derivative financing techniques enabled the packaging of subprime mortgages into collateralized debt obligations (CDO), in effect increasingly delinked from other asset-backed securities except RMBS and presented differently to different investors according to their tolerances for risk. Credit default swaps (CDS) appeared to defray some of the risk because CDS sellers put little capital into the process, but this in reality massively amplified the risk. The size of the CDS market in 2007 was more than US$61 trillion – at a time when entire the global value of stocks traded was running at US$88.4 trillion (Bank for International Settlements, 2020; World Bank, 2020).

Turning to the GCC, the dominant narrative begins 31 December 2019 when the Wuhan Municipal Health Commission in China reported to the World Health Organization that they had discovered 44 patients with pneumonia of unknown etiology. As soon as the COVID-19 virus was identified as the cause of the disease, almost all news and commentary sources attributed the source to the global trade in wild animals, although the evidence still has not been not conclusive. The focus was on wet markets – the evidence is also dubious here – and to the Wuhan wet market in particular, although there are now credible hypotheses that this location was a place of spreading and not necessarily the source of the pandemic.

Similar to the GFC, the GCC quickly lifted the embodied placement of disease transmission into the more abstract national and global realm as fixed points in a matrix of epidemiological statistics.

This growing database was then either used directly to drive national policies or skewed to make global comparisons in accordance with different political positions. Even an ignorant national populist leader like Donald Trump was forced to turn to scientific statistics to assert that the United States was supposedly 'doing well'. In his famous 2020 speech in the Rose Garden of the White House, the US President suggested that his compatriots should be proud of the 'fact' that 'the fatality rate has fallen 85% since April. Our excess mortality has been considerably lower than comparable countries' (Trump, 2020). It made no difference to Trump that a more nuanced analysis completely discounted the meaning of his way of presenting those two data-lines. Moreover, it did not seem to matter to his supporters that their President did not mention on the day of the speech that the world had just passed one million deaths, with most of those deaths occurring in the United States, Brazil, India, and Mexico. But what is most telling for our argument is the glaring disjuncture between the embodied experience of the crisis and the abstract framing of it. Even Donald Trump, one of the most populist-oriented politicians of our time, was forced to turn – even if selectively – to epidemiological statistics to make his case. And after his Rose Garden speech, the moment had passed to challenge those statistics for the next day as another wave of Covid statistics washed over the United States and the rest of the world.

The second most stricken country, Brazil, seems on the face of it to represent an exception to this disjuncture between embodied placement and abstracted relations insofar as President Jair Bolsonaro based his government's health policy vis-à-vis the pandemic on clear-cut epidemiological denialism without trying to employ statistics to bolster his arguments. However, it seems, as Francisco Ortega and Michael Orsini (2020) suggest, that Bolsonaro's denial of the consequences of COVID-19 was willfully and knowingly based on a standoff between the state and civil society that locked the President into a protracted battle for political legitimacy against civil health experts. While we might never find out what he personally believed, it is clear that politics dictated that he could not afford to agree with his opponents.

In summary, then, just as buying a house before the GFC remained an intimate activity *at one level*, contracting the coronavirus in 2020 remained an intimate condition for those whose bodies were affected, as well as their careers and loved ones. However, at the same time, and with more consequence and impact, these embodied relations were either lifted into the disembodied technical realm of mortality accounting or were distorted by populist politicians in a process that Achille Mbembe (2019) has called 'necropolitics': the use of political and economic power to manage human populations through their exposure to death. This tension between embodied placement and abstracted relations, we argue, belongs to the category of disjunctures that are likely to strengthen in our post-Covid world, thus intensifying the evolving social dynamics in our era of the Great Unsettling.

The disjuncture between embodied economic power and abstracted power

Using the same methodological framework of levels of embodied-to-disembodied relationality, the two crises confirmed a long-term relative shift of power, including the crucial capacities of transnational mobility and accumulation of wealth. During the GFC – a period defined by curtailing capital liquidity, while national governments worked hard to enhance global financial flows – significant counter-pressures came from many governments to slow the flows of migrants (Fix et al., 2009). So far, observed tendencies during the GCC have not been different: embodied movement is the most curtailed of any form of mobility. Although both crises have been described as democratizing their adverse effects across the world's population, a fine-grained conjunctural analysis applied to the case of wealth accumulation suggests a counter-narrative that is equally compelling. There has been an exacerbation of the division between rich and poor, an intensification of precarity, and a continuing privileging of those who are able to shift their means of power to more dematerialized assets, including financial power. This abstraction of economic power has over the last decades translated back into both enhanced material wealth (or not) and embodied wellbeing (or not), and the Global Covid Crisis appears to be no exception.

Once again, the United States and Brazil work well as comparative cases because of their complexity and their differences. In relation to the middle classes of both countries, their situations have been split. In the United States it is very clearly the case that those people who have added to their day-to-day activity of going to work the abstracted power of controlling dematerialized assets such as stocks have done much better than those who rely on pay-as-you-earn salaries. This explains the concerns about the crisis of the middle class. The geography of poverty is even more intense. In the United States, people whose homes were being repossessed found themselves confirmed as part of a localized, relatively immobilized 'precariat' (Standing, 2018). Indeed, we now know that the subprime mortgage consequences were focused on certain cohorts of people, not just localities. In the US it was predominantly Black and Hispanic residents who were evicted (Mayer & Pence, 2008).

Has this knowledge led policy-makers and lenders to transform positively the structural conditions of this problem? Quite the opposite. For example, the enduring practice of 'redlining' – the rejection of loans in red-lined zones on the basis of racial categories – was given even more abstracted power by the GFC. Mortgage redlining, prohibited by the US 1968 Fair Housing Act, has continued in the form of credit-profiling linked to algorithmically defined risk and to risk-based pricing. Thus, in effect, prohibited practices of redlining continue through abstracting its embodied meaning: 'a process of quantification in which non-quantitative information is translated into quantitative information, and subjective information becomes objectified in order to enable lenders to deal with individuals as risks' (Aalbers, 2007, p. 185). The home-ownership gap between Caucasians and African Americans is now wider than it was during the bygone era of legal color-based discrimination when embodied difference was treated as a basis for offering a mortgage or not.

In Brazil, the story is much the same, though for very different reasons. Overall home-ownership has declined since 2000 and inequalities have continued to increase. Brazilian records are not easy to access, but, in broad terms, a sense of the discrepancy can be illustrated by the simple figure that approximately 1% of the country's population own nearly 50% of the land, with an additional 36% state-owned.

The same structural inequalities can be seen in relation to the Global Covid Crisis. As one group of researchers concluded from the figures for the first three months of the crisis, US counties that are have large Black populations – that is, nearly 20% of all counties – accounted for 52% of Covid-related deaths nationally (Millett et al., 2020). In Brazil, Black workers, particularly those in the informal economy, were more likely to be exposed to the coronavirus. Despite universal access to health-care services through a Unified Health System (*Sisteme Único de Saúde*), recent practices of underfunding health care and neoliberal pressures to privatize health services, have led to profound inequalities, most profoundly reflected in significantly higher COVID-19 mortality rates for the poor. For example, the death rate from a confirmed infection was as high as 30.8% in Rio de Janeiro's Mare neighbourhood – a tangle of favelas on the city's north side – while it remained at only 2.4% in Leblon, an up-market beach district (Ortego & Orsini, 2020, 1,269).

Once again, our analysis of the tension between embodied economic power and mediated power suggests an exacerbation of the ongoing dynamics of the Great Unsettling.

Final reflections

In this essay, we have argued that the most likely mid-term prognosis for the world is an intensification of tensions and disjunctures that lead to a further strengthening of the complex dynamics we have called the Great Unsettling. This means that positive social transformations and deep political cooperation will be needed in order to build a more sustainable and socially just future. Positive transformation will not come on the wings of crises in themselves. As the world looks now, positive transformation will only come through a slow and uneven process of responding directly to the forms of ontological unsettling we laid out in this essay. Our discussion has focused on two crucial disjunctures, but we could only engage these tensions in an introductory way. A more comprehensive treatment of our subject would require analyzing additional disjunctures common to both the GFC and GCC.

One additional disjuncture, for example, concerns the way in which the responses to the crises were divided between treating them as an overgeneralized whole or as discrete problems. In particular, the governance of the crises was stretched between framing them as comprehensive, encompassing global events and managing them through discrete, technically measured, and institutionalized procedures (Langley, 2015). In another disjuncture, responses to technical experts during both crises were divided between giving experts working in narrowly construed disciplines too much power while denigrating others as variously irrelevant, alarmist or fake-news purveyors. In neither case has there been any sustained discussion of what each crisis meant for the optimal way of managing contested expertise or how different kinds of disciplinary input might be synthesized, including the relation between quantitative and qualitative evidence. Qualitative analysis tended to be neglected in both crises.

In a third additional disjuncture, both crises revealed that the nature of work has continued to be divided between a more demanding personal experience of expressive commitment to the workplace – stronger for intellectual and service work than for manual and technical work – and a more abstracted, intensely applied set of surveillance and performance measures – similarly intense but differently configured across the various kinds of labour. The move to remote work and remote workforce management during the GCC has accelerated rather than transformed what has been a longer-term process that includes both global offshoring and current reshoring efforts.

Taken together, these social disjunctures have had incongruous effects. They add to a deep unsettling, both locally and globally, but without this leading to positive transformation. Despite, the rich epidemiological analysis of the Global Covid Crisis and the recognition of poverty and racism as major causes of higher mortality rates, there has been little or no remaking of the priorities of health systems and their social contexts around the world. This parallels the GFC. Despite comprehensive and public critical analysis of this earlier crisis and the recognition of uneven economic vulnerability, the '1 per cent' have continued to get disproportionately richer. To reinforce but one example discussed earlier, it should be especially noted how the global spreading of financial risk before and after the GFC has been associated with a further abstraction of the instruments for managing value – ostensibly to allay 'local' risk. This had the opposite effect of containing risk – both elaborating the scale of the risk and condensing the time-scale in which it occurs (Bryan & Rafferty, 2014). This process is akin to the way in which hedging shifted from a risk-management process for agriculture – namely, to stabilize prices in relation to forthcoming seasonal variations – to a new form of intense speculation.

Indeed, both modalities of financialization are part of the Great Unsettling to the extent that they stretch and destabilize the relationship between the meaning of 'value' and the 'cost' of material objects or processes: houses, wheat, corn, and even securing against bad weather. Like agricultural hedging, the process of securing against local or national mortgage risk, turned a half-century of innovation into its opposite, namely, a way of speculating by using the instruments of risk-management. The growing disjuncture between embodied placed materiality and abstracted fiduciary value magnified risk exponentially and thus served as a core driver of the crisis. Despite the bailouts and some changed governance measures after the GFC, nothing has changed to mitigate this disjuncture.

Finally, let us return to our domain descriptions of the unsettling to suggest what could be done to respond to different structural conditions of the two crises. First, *ecologically*, if technoscientific interventions into nature – setting up conditions of hyper-exploitation and instrumentalizing nature as a resource – has been the cause of a number of crises from the Sixth Extinction to increased zoonotic pathogen-transfer including COVID-19, then we should expect a new attention to this question? The lack of discussion of this basic concern throughout the GCC, even though it is directly relevant to zoonotic transfer, is not a source of hope. Challenging and curtailing technoscientific interventions into nature is imperative.

Second, *economically*, if derivative instruments for abstracting value are wrenching the relation between risk-management and 'the real economy', then should not we expect focused attention on reforming financial markets? While it is true that since the GFC securities like credit default swaps have declined, derivatives as a whole have increased from US$507 trillion in 2007 to US$640 trillion in 2019. Over the same period, globally traded stocks have declined from US$88.4 trillion to $60.3 trillion. Thus, we regrettably conclude that not much has changed here in the direction of positive social transformations. In fact, we are now facing similar risks to those we did more than a decade ago. The reforms to the financial market were minimal. In any case, beyond financial reform, more systematic attention, we suggest, should be paid to the structural causes of the crises in question and what should be done about the cleaving outcomes. In the case of finance, it cannot be simply a matter of banning derivatives because the relation between rapacious speculation and virtuous risk-management has now become both unsettled *and* blurred. They are bound up together within contemporary financial capitalism for good *and* ill (Bryan & Rafferty, 2006). This suggests that, far beyond managing the excesses of capitalism, radically decentering capitalism as the dominant mode of production and exchange will be necessary.

Third, *politically*, if disruptions to the meaning and practice of political representation are confirming longer-term profound assaults on basic understandings of good governance, then should not this deepening problem of a legitimation crisis be squarely confronted? For example, public trust in government in the United States has fallen from 77% in 1964 to 17% in 2019. (Pew Research Center, 2019). Most countries around the world show similar declines, albeit not quite as steep as for the US. Part of the problem is that people are still so completely caught in short-term electoral questions over who will govern that we have little capacity to take on this fundamental issue in a sustained way. This entails fundamentally reforming democratic processes.

Indeed, this problem is compounded as the nature of twenty-first-century global problems is itself being used by populists around the world to fight electoral battles. It connects to the fourth domain of cultural unsettling. If relativizing and deconstructing social meaning has not proved to be the liberatory force that its proponents projected – and that covers the entire ideological spectrum from the poststructuralist Left to the populist Right – then shouldn't we be seeking an alternative grounding for meaning that goes beyond either highly individualized belief, mediated (and manipulated) by the social media or positivistic statistical measurement? This ontological challenge is perhaps the most difficult problem of all. Unless and until we make progress on that front, we are in for stormy weather with little prospect of finding a safe harbour that provides shelter from the intensifying unsettling of our global-local nexus.

Note

1. These changes can be understood as explicable in the coming together of the exponential shifts described in terms of the Great Acceleration (Steffen et al. 2015), and the disjunctive consequences of the Great Unsettling.

Disclosure statement

No potential conflict of interest was reported by the author(s).

ORCID

Paul James ⓘ http://orcid.org/0000-0002-8591-4594
Manfred B. Steger ⓘ http://orcid.org/0000-0002-1679-6539

References

Aalbers, M. (2007). *Place, exclusion, and mortgage markets*. Blackwell.
Aalbers, M. (2009). Geographies of the financial crisis. *Area*, *41*(1), 34–42. https://doi.org/10.1111/j.1475-4762.2008.00877.x
Arvidsson, A. (2016). Facebook and finance: On the social logic of the derivative. *Theory, Culture & Society*, *33*(6), 3–23. https://doi.org/10.1177/0263276416658104
Bank for International Settlements. (2020). Retrieved November 4, 2020, from www.bis.org
Bryan, D., & Rafferty, M. (2006). *Capitalism with derivatives: A political economy of financial derivatives, capital and class*. Palgrave Macmillan.
Bryan, D., & Rafferty, M. (2014). Financial derivatives as social policy beyond crisis. *Sociology*, *48*(5), 887–903. https://doi.org/10.1177/0038038514539061
Fix, M., Papademetriou, D. G., Batalova, J., Terrazas, A., Yi-Ying Lin, S., & Mittelstadt, M. (2009). *Migration and the global recession: A report commissioned by the BBC world service*. Migration Policy Institute.
Gramsci, A. (1971). *Selections from the prison notebooks*. International Publishers.
Habermas, J. (1988). *Legitimation crisis*. Polity Press. (Original work published 1973)

James, P. (2020). Global cities as mediated spaces: The role of media in forming contradictory places. In Z. Krajina & D. Stevenson (Eds.), *Routledge companion to urban media and communication* (pp. 174–184). Routledge.

Langley, P. (2015). *Liquidity lost: The governance of the global financial crisis*. Oxford University Press.

Livesay, F. (2017). *From global to local: The making of things and the end of globalization*. Vintage.

Mandal, A., Roy, R., Ghosh, D., Dhaliwal, S. S., Toor, A. S., Mukhopadhyay, S., & Majumder, A. (2020). COVID-19 Pandemic: Sudden restoration in global environmental quality and its impact on climate change. Eneraxiv preprint. Retrieved June 22, 2020, from http://www.enerarxiv.org/thesis/1589672734.pdf

Mayer, C. J., & Pence, K. (2008). *Subprime mortgages: What, where and to whom?* (Working Paper 14083). National Bureau of Economic Research.

Mbembe, A. (2019). *Necro-politics*. Duke University Press.

McKibben, B. (1989). *The end of nature*. Bloomsbury.

McLuhan, M. (1994). *Understanding media: The extensions of man*. MIT Press.

Millett, G. A., Jones, A. T., Benkeser, D., Baral, S., Mercer, L., Beyrer, C., Honermann, B., Lankiewicz, E., Mena, L., Crowley, J. S., Sherwood, J., & Sullivan, P. S. (2020). Assessing differential impacts of COVID-19 on black communities. *Annals of Epidemiology, 47*, 37–44. https://doi.org/10.1016/j.annepidem.2020.05.003

Nesvetailova, A. (2007). *Fragile finance: Debt, speculation and crisis in the age of global credit*. Palgrave-Macmillan.

Ortega, F., & Orsini, M. (2020). Governing COVID-19 without government in Brazil: Ignorance, neoliberal authoritarianism, and the collapse of public health leadership. *Global Public Health, 15*(9), 1257–1277. https://doi.org/10.1080/17441692.2020.1795223

Peters, G., Marland, G., Le Quéré, C., Boden, T., Canadell, J. G., & Raupach, M. R. (2012). Rapid growth in CO_2 emissions after the 2008–2009 global financial crisis. *Nature Climate Change, 2*(1), 2–4. https://doi.org/10.1038/nclimate1332

Pew Research Center. (2019). Public trust in government, 1958–2019. Retrieved November 12, 2020, from https://www.pewresearch.org/politics/2019/04/11/public-trust-in-government-1958-2019/

Polanyi, K. (1944). *The great transformation: The political and economic origins of our time*. Beacon Press.

Read, C. (2009). *Global financial meltdown: How we can avoid the next economic crisis*. Palgrave-Macmillan.

Robinson, W. I. (2020). *The global police state*. Pluto Press.

Standing, G. (2018). The precariat: Today's transformative class? *Development, 61*(1-4), 115–121. https://doi.org/10.1057/s41301-018-0182-5

Steffen, W., Broadgate, W., Deutsch, L., Gaffney, O., & Ludwig, C. (2015). The trajectory of the anthropocene: The great acceleration. *The Anthropocene Review, 2*(1), 81–98. https://doi.org/10.1177/2053019614564785

Steger, M. B., & James, P. (2019). *Globalization matters: Engaging the global in unsettled times*. Cambridge University Press.

Steger, M. B., & James, P. (2020). Disjunctive globalization: COVID-19, capitalism and the great unsettling. *Theory, Culture and Society, 37*(7-8), 1–17. https://doi.org/10.1177/0263276420957744

Tooze, A. (2019). *Crashed: How a decade of financial crisis changed the world*. Penguin Books.

Trump, D. (2020, September 28). Rose Garden speech. Retrieved November 7, 2020, from www.whitehouse.gov/briefings-statements/remarks-president-trump-update-nations-coronavirus-testing-strategy/

Vandevelde, M., Rennison, J., Campbell, C., Bernard, S., & Manibog, C. (2018, September 5). The story of a house: How private equity swooped in after the subprime crisis. *Financial Times*. Retrieved November 4, 2020, from https://ig.ft.com/story-of-a-house/

Varoufakis, Y. (2011). *The global minotaur: America, the true origins of the financial crisis and the future of the world economy*. Zed Books.

Wodak, J. (2020). (Human-inflected) evolution in an age of (human-induced) extinction: Synthetic biology meets the anthropocene. *Humanities, 9*(4), 126. https://doi.org/10.3390/h9040126

World Bank. (2020). https://data.worldbank.org/indicator/CM.MKT.TRAD.CD

Wright, R. (2020, March 17). There's an unlikely beneficiary of coronavirus: The planet. *CNN Hong Kong*. Retrieved June 22, 2020, from https://edition.cnn.com/2020/03/16/asia/china-pollution-coronavirus-hnk-intl/index.html

Global transitioning: beyond the Covid-19 pandemic

James H. Mittelman

ABSTRACT
Picking up on Fernand Braudel's schematic of three speeds of time, this article examines the overlapping periods of vaccine nationalism, viral globalization, and runaway capitalism: running away, meaning a lack of effective regulatory controls and lax democratic accountability. The stark contradiction between vaccine nationalism and a planetary health crisis propels this unfolding of history. The two tendencies feed one another, affording an opportunity to grasp the flow of history and the system's fragility. This dynamic highlights the conundrum of equitable distribution of the drug on a world level. It draws attention to the imperative of replacing vaccine nationalism with a global vaccine ethics based on rectitude and social justice. This complex offers an opportunity to restructure the world in ways that are accountable, inclusive, and protective of the common good. In this way, Braudelian historicism is deployed to chart an avenue of inquiry about transitioning to a better world order.

When the Covid-19 pandemic pulled back the curtain on globalized capitalism and its transformations, vexing questions arose: What does it reveal about the kinds of transformation the contagion unleashed, and what does it tell us about harbingers of future world order?

Clearly, the international system has been unable to ensure worldwide access to vaccines and the supply of related products to fight the corona disease. It has failed to respond decisively to a global pandemic, which, by definition, transcends national borders. This spawns a related question, how to serve the public good in the face of national restrictions on exports of vaccine-making drugs and thwart the virus?

By and large, scientists of the world have performed admirably in discovering an effective vaccine. Their epistemic communities have produced ground-breaking knowledge on how to build capacity to address the worldwide crisis in global health. Yet politicians have been slow or resistant to find ways to transcend their national jurisdictions and relax the strictures of sovereignty. Weak political institutions have hampered a resolute international response to the deadly disease.

When the coronavirus pandemic recedes broadly and restrictions on human interactions are minimized, a transition toward a post-pandemic world will begin. In the past, deadly viruses have not suddenly disappeared.[1] Like prior pandemics such as polio and HIV/AIDS, Covid-19 will stutter along, even though subject to preventative protocols and controls, and continue to endanger public health. History shows that pandemics can reignite in serial form. Known as post-polio syndrome, outbreaks of polio, for example, reappear from time to time. By necessity, humans will need to live with the coronavirus risk.

To understand transformations in a temporal sense, the economic historian Fernand Braudel provides insights into the grand tradition of the Annales school. He offers a way of thinking about the churning of history at three speeds. One is a rapid time scale. This is *l'histoire événementielle*, the short-time span experienced in daily life, which is the métier of journalists and policy specialists (Braudel, 1980, pp. 27–28; Cox, 1995; Heilleiner, 1997). Next, the medium-term, the conjunctural perspective, corresponds to cycles and rhythms that may take a decade, a quarter century, 50 years, or even longer (1980, pp. 29–30). Third, in his magnum opus (1996), Braudel chronicles the *longue durée*. In this deeply-rooted and decentred history, Braudel evokes a tempo in slow motion, almost imperceptible, verging on inertia (1980, p. 33; also see Braudel, 1977). This segment of history emphasizes deep social structures and thick descriptions.

Ranging from micro time to structural time, Braudelian historicism can be employed as both a heuristic and dialectic to analyse the shift to a post-pandemic world. Braudel's intellectual toolbox facilitates mobilizing history and designing just futures.

Correspondingly, this article examines the time frames of vaccine nationalism, viral globalization, and runaway globalization: running away, meaning a lack of effective regulatory controls and lax democratic accountability. These periods overlap with tensions among the three phases. The first two periods bracket a liminal phase, a precursor to the third: a still evolving, historical structure. Capitalist dynamics are central to this unfolding of history.

In what follows, my message is threefold. First, within Braudel's time frames, there is a stark contradiction between vaccine nationalism and the planetary health crisis. In this dialectic, the two tendencies feed one another, affording opportunities to grasp the flow of history and the evolving system's fragility. In fact, there is ample opportunity to build capacity, global cooperation, and resilience. Second, the development of an effective vaccine leads to the mostly unheeded call for *equitable distribution* of the drug on a world level, a contested matter with myriad proposed remedies.

Third, this draws attention to the imperative of replacing vaccine nationalism with a global vaccine ethics based on rectitude and social justice. In a Polanyian sense, the ethics of democratic globalization turn on re-embedding the economy in society. And in Gramscian terms, it is about building counterhegemony: an order that is tolerant of differences; seeks new ways to accommodate them in an open, participatory manner; and embraces a dispersion of power. The goal is to inculcate a new moral order in lieu of the dominant ethics – currently an ethos of efficiency, competition, individualism, and consumption inscribed in neoliberalism.[2] This pressure, in turn, challenges policymakers and sparks attendant debates in the public square.

Another objective in this article is to imagine a way to map and shape the forces coming into play in superseding the coronavirus crisis. It would cut against common-sense thinking about the pandemic and discard the formative influences of reigning paradigms. Let us now probe the three overlapping timelines, beginning with vaccine nationalism.

The history of events: vaccine nationalism

In November 2020, drugmakers announced a breakthrough in discovering a highly effective vaccine for preventing Covid-19. Rival firms were not far behind the frontrunners in their efforts to thwart the global coronavirus pandemic. But vexing questions about widespread distribution had yet to be resolved.

The problems run deep. In the face of warnings about the risk of a pandemic, power holders' lack of foresight was egregious. A workable strategy for mitigating the pandemic requires anticipatory knowledge and a strategy for clearing the political and economic blockage that stymies relief.

Nonetheless, this issue is typically seen as a biomedical challenge, a matter of producing a successful vaccine. It should instead be understood more comprehensively as a *trifecta of science, politics, and profit*.

This perspective reflects my experience aboard a flight from Entebbe, Uganda, a hotspot for the HIV/AIDS pandemic. Seated next to me was the head of the Infectious Diseases Institute, part of the School of Medicine at Makerere University in Kampala, Uganda. Asked about prospects for stopping the pandemic, the doctor who, like me, had been living and working in Kampala for years, replied, 'The interesting research is being done in your field, the social sciences, not mine. We are trying to understand why people do what they do.'

He had in mind the empirical findings of medical geographers and cultural anthropologists. They demonstrate that the HIV/AIDS infection rate soared along routes established by the slave trade and subsequently frequented by drivers trucking across borders, providing a robust market for sex workers. The incidence of the disease varied markedly among Uganda's monogamous and polygamous societies, the ones that practice circumcision and others that do not, religious communities, and ethnicities, as well as by income and educational levels. Social research also delved deeply into other political and economic structures that help explain the disparate incidence of this condition. A major factor is that millions of people – not only in Uganda – distrust public authorities and suspect that expert advice is tainted by self-serving politicians and dubious evidence.

To be sure, reining in the worldwide corona calamity requires coming to grips with human behaviour, wrapped up with money and power. The hospitalization of a Covid-positive US president, Donald Trump, a science-denier bent on beating competitor nations in a race to bring a vaccine to market, betrays this challenge.

The 2020 pandemic recession and its consequences are rooted in market failure and malgovernance. As early as 2011, the World Health Organization warned about the need to prepare for coming pandemics and their potentially huge toll (Velásquez, 2020, p. 1). In 2015 and 2016, Bill Gates, a business magnate, software entrepreneur, and philanthropist, similarly told policymakers, including incoming President Trump, to prepare to respond to an infectious-disease pandemic (Bill Gates warns of epidemic that could kill over 30 million people, 2017, p. 4). Unquestionably, there was and is a sense of urgency about this threat. Nonetheless, the Trump administration dismissed Gates's advice. For their part, giant drug companies proceeded to invest substantially in products that turn a quick profit rather than on long-term R&D.

The Bill and Melinda Gates Foundation, the world's largest private philanthropy, a $50 billion operation, is winning plaudits for its vision and willingness to plow money into the race to deliver a corona vaccine to multitudes. This philanthropy substitutes for or, some believe, complements governmental efforts to safeguard public health. But make no mistake about the forces behind Gates' move. The foundation does not act solely out of altruism. Rather than representing charitable giving, the resources granted emanate from both genuine concern for the victims of a lethal disease and strategic acumen at accumulating capital.

Philanthropic capitalism encompasses profit making by a funder that receives huge earnings from its investments, guided by wealth managers, pricey accountants, and consultants who small enterprises can ill afford.[3] In the United States, philanthropies are subject to a low spend rate, required by federal authorities, and benefit from their status as tax-exempt nonprofit organizations.

The South Centre, an intergovernmental organization based in Geneva, reports that five transnational corporations account for around 80 per cent of global vaccine sales (Velásquez, 2020, p. 3). In the chase for an effective vaccine and antiviral therapies, owners of stocks in big pharma have gained handsomely from exclusive licensing, monopoly pricing, taxpayer-financed emergency sub-sidies, guaranteed purchase contracts, and clauses in the contracts that provide immunity from liability if anything goes awry. In the American case, the terms of drug makers' vaccine contracts with the federal government are shrouded in secrecy. Despite calls for disclosure, transparency, and accountability, the records, as a matter of companies' policies, are not released. It is unknown whether political connections, cronyism, and price gouging are in play. There's no reliable evidence about the kinds of deals that affluent countries and giant pharmaceuticals have cut.

Mistakenly, a Belgian official disclosed a price list, which indicates that US taxpayers paid $19.50 per dose whereas the corresponding charge for Europeans was $14.70 (Apuzzo & Gebrekidan, 2021). The European Commission negotiated a price of $2.19 per dose of the vaccine produced by the University of Oxford and AstraZeneca, while South Africa paid more than twice that amount for the same product (Apuzzo & Gebrekidan, 2021). Some of the poorest countries have yet to be able to negotiate deals. Strikingly, uneven market conditions are protecting companies, leaving marginalized communities unprotected, and costing millions of lives. Let us now look at sub-sequent periods and parse the ways that these issues are interwoven.

Intermediate-term conjunctures: viral globalization

The three 'As' – availability, access, and affordability – warrant further scrutiny, public debate, and policy making in a democratic manner. With large drug companies competing against one another, the contestants insist on keeping critical information on scientific breakthroughs under wraps. Wary of stealth and emulation, they secure data by classifying it as protected intellectual property. These are the rules of the corporate, state-sanctioned game. Left to taken-for-granted modi oper-andi, the three 'As' are treated as business as usual. But these issues turn on the inconvenient ques-tions of who is empowered to decide on them and who authorizes the decision makers.

(1) *Availability*: When Jonas Salk introduced the polio vaccine, he was asked who owned the patent. Dr Salk responded: 'The people, I would say. There is no patent. You might as well ask, could you patent the sun?' (as quoted in Chowdhury & Jomo, 2020). This was before the adoption of rules for ownership of intellectual property rights under the World Trade Organization (WTO) and antecedent agreements.

(2) *Access*: Globally, who should be at the front of the line to be vaccinated against future mutations of the virus? The countries where the pharmaceuticals that first produce the vaccine are headquartered? But in other locales where the pathogen is raging, how long will it take to build the capability to ramp up supply chains for the general public and not primarily the rich? In the United States, the Food and Drug Administration gave priority to health care workers and other vulnerable groups. But why should people in a vulnerable age bracket be entitled to lifesaving vaccines when others such as members of minority communities are disproportio-nately harmed by the contagion and are not so privileged?

(3) *Affordability*: Big pharma weighs heavily in determining the cost of a vaccine, mostly levied on citizens as taxation. The poor in affluent countries and the masses in impoverished countries are least able to gain timely, affordable access. Research shows that uneven distribution of the drug within and among countries deepens global divides (Çakmakh et al., 2021). By the time that the wealthy countries had pre-purchased most of the supply of the vaccine, many countries in the global South would still have to wait until 2024 or later. In light of reliance on global supply and production chains, as well as on other economic flows such as cross-border

trade and foreign investment, rich countries have acted against their own interests. Until supplier countries substantially recover from the pandemic, the rest of the world's production capacity will remain diminished. At this writing (July 2021), the developed economies bear up to 53 per cent of the global economic costs of the pandemic even when they reach a high-level vaccination rate for their own populations (Çakmakh et al., 2021, p. 1). A large part of the underlying problem is that the representatives of marginalized communities have not been invited to the high table where crucial decisions about the three 'As' are hammered out.

The rapid spread of the virus prompted policymakers and researchers to search for a way out of these conundrums. They have encountered a formidable hurdle: the ongoing tension between a planetary health crisis and vaccine nationalism. Infectious diseases don't respect territorial borders. A global pandemic necessitates a global response. By themselves, fragmented national and subnational policies cannot sufficiently control international mobility and transnational flows. This disorderly hierarchy has established a highly skewed distribution of vaccines.

According to a Duke University database, governments had purchased 7 billion vaccine doses by January 2021 (Duke Global Health Institute, 2021). By that time, high-income countries had obtained 4.2 billion of them and held 60 per cent of the global supply, yet represented only 16 per cent of the world population (2021). In June 2021, Tedros Adanom Ghebreyesus, Director-General of the World Health Organization, reported that 44 per cent of doses had been administered in richer countries. In poorer nations, the figure is just 0.4 per cent (as quoted in United Nations, 2021). Drawing on other sources, Carlos Correa, executive director of the South Centre, notes that while 85 per cent of vaccine administered worldwide had been in high- and upper-middle-income countries, only 1 per cent of inoculations were administered in low-income countries (2021). Added to this unevenness, some well-to-do countries' supply of drugs far exceeds their populations. The EU countries, for instance, have enough doses for 6.6 times their population; the US, 5; Canada, 12; the UK, 8; and Australia, 7 (Chowdhury & Jomo, 2021).

The remedy for stemming a deadly disease that transgresses borders calls for two-track collaboration: multilateralism pressured by civil society organizations. The route is to summon the political will to achieve global coordination. The drivers come from above and below: elected policymakers pressed by social movements that spur collective action. Many of the latter have entreated the former to support India and South Africa's proposal at the WTO for temporary waivers on the protection of certain intellectual property rights during the Covid-19 pandemic. In parallel, civil society must build public trust and strive for shared ends. This path is clearly demarcated. Social justice activists are attempting to provide the impetus. Their messaging has to be clear. Galvanizing narratives about equitable distribution of the vaccine have the potential to generate widespread support.

Inclusivity is key to equitable access, distribution, and cost. A plausible way to achieve this goal is on the table. Access to Covid-19 Tools (ACT) Accelerator is a proposal under consideration by the Group of 20 nations for combating the pandemic. It centres on promoting global cooperation to reduce the spread of the Covid disease. Given that wealthy countries had hurriedly purchased supplies of the leading vaccine candidates, limiting inventories for poor countries, ACT is an effort to obtain waivers on proprietary rights, share knowledge, and transfer technology. A principal obstacle is insufficient funding, estimated at US$31.3 billion in 2021, to secure 2 billion vaccine doses, treatments, and the availability of enough tests to throttle the pandemic. The imperative is to fill the gap between pledges and actual contributions.

The Covid-19 Vaccines Global Access (COVAX) facility complements ACT. It is supported by the WTO, and partners with nongovernmental organizations and drug manufacturers for establishing ethically sound distribution of the vaccine at the world level. To combat the pandemic, COVAX aims to guard against misallocation, foster transparency, and treat vaccines as a global public good. In a globalized era marked by transnational mobility, the distribution of the drug will create a handful of national safe havens. But the peril lies in adopting unjust principles that severely hurt the poorest countries and risk reinfection.

To avoid paying this high price, more than 190 countries have signed non-binding commitment agreements to join the COVAX initiative. These accords pool resources for all partnering states to ward off the pandemic. Still, these agreements require staunch will and additional funding.

Without an adequate amount of doses to vaccinate the entire world population in the near future, corporate control over supply is bound to impede quelling the contagion. Fundamentally, this is a matter of how capitalist globalization works. Impoverished countries cannot compete in the open market. A my-country-first strategy along with a market-based approach to the pandemic is the heart of the problem. As matters stand, several poor countries will continue to be left three years behind to fully vaccinate their populations.

Most rich countries and large corporations have taken the position that they funded and undertook the cutting-edge research, manufacturing, and development of the vaccines. Their proponents say that citizens of these nations should therefore have preferential access for the life-saving inoculations. The drug companies' champions also claim that sharing their proprietary knowledge with the rest of the world would jeopardize innovation and discourage further vaccine research. Opposition to the temporary suspension of the WTO's Agreement on Trade-Related Aspects of Intellectual Property Rights, with its compulsory licensing provisions, is based on these grounds. Bill Gates and others contend, too, that developing countries lack the means and ability to produce the vaccine safely.

On the other side of this debate, prolocutors argue that possession of wealth does not justify exclusive rights to control the supply of life-saving drugs. From this standpoint, it is a myth that incentives and new products arise primarily because of competition in the marketplace. Instead, information should be freely shared in the public interest. These critics hold that the pharmaceuticals' advocates and allies are upholding the industry's self-serving position and realizing superprofits. In fact, developing countries have previously produced vaccines – the Serum Institute of India is one of the largest vaccine manufacturers in the world – and should not be constrained by rules on international property rights.

Saddled by a skyrocking rate of corona infections, India halted exporting its vaccines in 2021 in order to meet its own needs. Important, too, the market system has provided opportunities for both the tech industry and surveillance companies to gather data and expand their businesses because of what is regarded as the exceptionalism of the coronavirus pandemic. In public discourse, these circumstances are often referred to as 'unprecedented' and 'unparalleled'. But there is ample precedent for the current pandemic, including the Black Plague, Spanish influenza, and HIV-AIDS.

From a political perspective, the contemporary Italian philosopher Giorgio Ambagen warns that the state of exception, introduced by the sovereign as an emergency measure, is easily transposed into the rule (Agamben, 1999, p. 162). With the force of law, it can become a normal condition, restraining freedom and used to justify authoritarianism.

As the virus mutates, there is the danger that new variants will dodge the vaccine. Likely, the disease will continually circulate and infect individual bodies. Contact tracing, thoroughgoing testing, and other such measures serve to legitimize surveillance. Moreover, the war against the virus targets citizens themselves. An invisible enemy is within us and engaged in civil war (Agamben, 2020b). Rooted in market capitalism, this warfare breeds ethical failings and sacrifices moral principles (Agamben, 2020a).

The longue durée: runaway capitalism

Amid the profound changes and despair noted above, the world is approaching a post-pandemic age. The transition marks a slow-moving, profound shift. After a time of restrictions on human mobility, this churn is a period of runaway capitalism.

Both continuities and discontinuities with prior forms of capitalism are palpable. Post-pandemic, the driving forces will continue to be relentless competition and the expansive process of accumulation. To counter 'vaccine diplomacy' by Beijing and Moscow, members of the Group of Seven, a club of wealthy countries, plan to purchase 500 million doses of Covid-19 vaccines and distribute them in the global South. Some of the big pharmaceuticals had already agreed to ship large supplies of doses to impoverished countries on a non-profit basis.

Global competition is also on display among affluent national states – Britain versus European Union members – in trying to beat one another to garner a stock of coronavirus vaccines. But, as mentioned, most of these countries had already accumulated sizeable deliveries of doses through advance purchase agreements (Mueller & Stevis-Gridneff, 2021). In the global South, China and India, two countries with the capacity to export Covid vaccines, are locked in competition over distribution.

To contextualize, twenty-first-century capitalism in its several varieties is experiencing a triple transition from its antecedent forms.[4] Sketched out below, three trends constitute runaway capitalism. Each strand is emerging as a major feature of a post-pandemic world.

One of them is algorithmic capitalism, which is largely, though not entirely, driven by digital innovations. It embodies human and machine intelligence (O'Neil, 2016; Pasquale, 2015). So, too, algorithmic capitalism embraces numeric governance insofar as it objectifies indicators – for instance, of excellence, poverty, corruption, and good governance – and translates them into policy. In the political sphere and commerce, metrics encoded in machines are used to mobilize and allocate resources, roles heretofore played by elected officials.

The second is cognitive capitalism wherein the knowledge portion of commodities outstrips the physical components that produce them. In the cognitive architecture, intellectual capital is denominated as information and big data (Boutang, 2011; Fuchs, 2012; Mager, 2012; Peters & Bulut, 2011). Since knowledge is a source of economic growth, knowledge institutions, including universities, research networks, and applied training programmes, play an increasingly salient role in the evolution of capitalism. Accordingly, the composition of the workforce and labour-management relations undergo dramatic changes, as the gig economy shows.

Third, philanthropic capitalism is a market-based, for-profit approach to solving intractable problems such as poverty and environmental degradation. Seemingly softening the jagged edges of markets, it entails disbursing funds, often by wealthy individuals and families whose activities substitute for, or parallel, the legitimate role of the state. They determine which issues merit support and which ones do not allocate revenue to those favoured. Private foundations proceed with little public accountability or transparency, thereby sidestepping democratic principles of governance.

These trajectories – algorithmic, cognitive, and philanthropic capitalism – are integrally connected. There is no single determinant for all times and places. No one vector takes precedence. They interconnect not in a circular manner but as historically specific conditions warrant. These components are anchored in specific times and places. The three-fold designation allows for reciprocal actions among the elements.

In practice, they are converging in multiple ways. For example, algorithms, in conjunction with artificial intelligence (AI), are creating new opportunities for knowledge-intensive jobs. This development enters into funders' decisions about distributing grants for educational and research programmes. With mounting public disinvestment in higher education in numerous countries, philanthropies are an increasingly vital source of revenue for developing knowledge communities' projects on algorithms and AI. These disbursements ramp up both algorithmic capitalism and cognitive capitalism. The latter manifests in the growing share of knowledge in commodity production. A pivotal aspect of this pattern is philanthropic capital's predilection for assigning higher priority to projects that provide better indexes used as inputs for machine intelligence, and lower priority to concerns about traditional wage labour. Overlap among the three trajectories culminates in emerging coalescence among the elements of runaway capitalism.

In the foregoing discussion, I have sought to stretch a Braudelian framework by adding a fundamental category – resistance – and introduced granular data on the case of Covid-19. Expanding Braudelian historicism by giving explicit attention to this dimension of capitalism, pushback by myriad social forces, can enrich analysis.

An opportunity to reimagine the future

To round up my main points: In the current interregnum, three speeds of time are layered. Braudel's temporal modalities – the immediate moment, the medium term of a decade or decades, and the *longue durée* – are in play. From this perspective, a historical transition cannot be fully grasped if it primarily focuses on the here and now without looking at the long arc of history.

The time scale must extend to transformative developments. Braudel's variegated tableau emphasizes social conditions on the ground, including the spread of infectious diseases and their pathogenic agents. He paints a picture of the transmission of tuberculosis, malaria, sleeping sickness, and plague (Braudel, 1980, pp. 105–119).

Taking a cue from Braudel, a robust analysis of runaway capitalism covers the three time spans. It finds direct precursors in vaccine nationalism and the conjunctural period of viral globalization. In a more evolved form, a tripartite system is operative: the interlocking tendencies of algorithmic, cognitive, and philanthropic capitalism. To my mind, their confluence is integral to the coming order.

Conceptualizing this complex enables imagining a plural world order in ways that are accountable and inclusive. This is more of a potential than a set of lived practices. There would be several voices in this mix, sometimes at odds with one another; myriad visions; and no lack of concrete proposals. The conversation about future world order is a sign of vitality, a quest for a better community.

While the immediacy of the coronavirus and the pandemic recession are morbid symptoms of a confluence of crises in global capitalism, their lasting effects will pervade the *longue durée*. Meanwhile, the contagion of runaway capitalism wherein the rich get richer during worldwide health and environmental crises continues apace (Piketty, 2020). Even before Covid-19, deep-rooted problems in public health roiled many countries and endure. As noted, they have been greeted by nationalist policies that mandate hoarding drugs without a moral anchor.

Looking ahead to the aftermath of Covid-19, there will be valuable lessons to be learned. These lessons should beckon adaptation in stakeholders' own contexts and strive to be reliable, replicable, and scalable. This can help leverage global transformations toward democratic futures.

Ultimately, the motors of coming transformations will be countervailing power and alternative knowledge. Critical knowledge feeds on contesting ideas, putting them in practice, and, amid disinformation narratives, ensuring that the public sphere is open to evidence-based debate. Ultimately, the litmus of transformative ideas is their practical results.

Reflecting on global transitioning, Braudel maintains that '[h]istory is always begun anew; it is always working itself out, striving to surpass itself' (1977, p. 115). If there is indeed a new beginning, the global future remains to be shaped and reshaped. One hopes that the Covid-19 pandemic jolts humans to dare to journey down a path toward a safe and morally just order.

Notes

1. For background on pandemics before Covid-19, see Saker et al. (2004), Scholte (2005), and Aaltola (2020).
2. Velásquez, G. (2020). For proposed guidelines on equitable treatment of Covid-19, see Abbas (2020) and Hastings Center (2020)
3. The literature on philanthropic capitalism is voluminous. Matthew Bishop is often credited with coining the term. See 'The birth of philanthrocapitalism' (2006) and Bishop and Green (2009). But it actually appeared earlier in Bernholz (2004). According to Bishop, the philanthropic industry assumes the characteristics of a capitalist marketplace and turns philanthropists into investors. For Bishop and Green (2009), it involves the application of business methods to philanthropy. More critical perspectives focus on the ways in which the activities of foundations align with neoliberalism. These arguments may be found in McGoey (2015) and Reich (2018). Building on this work, Burns (2019, p. 1101) deems the coupling of philanthropy and capitalism as 'a new site for capital accumulation'.
4. The ensuing discussion of the three trends of runaway capitalism encapsulates a multi-year project that I am developing. The existing research, I find, is full of ambiguities and blind spots, but has vast potential for reinterpretation.

Acknowledgements

The author owes a debt of gratitude to Linda J. Yarr and this journal's anonymous reviewers for incisive comments on earlier drafts of this paper. And thanks to Frieder G. Dengler and Julie Radomski for stellar research assistance. The author is grateful to American University for supporting this work.

Disclosure statement

No potential conflict of interest was reported by the author.

References

Aaltola, M. (2020, March). *Covid-19 – a trigger for global transformation? Political distancing, global decoupling and growing distrust in health governance* (Working Paper no. 13). Finnish Institute of International Affairs.

Abbas, M. Z. (2020, November). *Practical implications of 'vaccine nationalism': A short-sighted and risky approach in response to COVID-19* (Research Paper 124). South Centre.

Agamben, G. (1999). *Potentialities: Collected essays in philosophy* (D. Heller-Rozman, Ed. and Trans.). Stanford University Press. (Original work published 1998)

Agamben, G. (2020a, April 14). *A question* (A. Kotsko, Trans.). https://itself.blog/2020/04/15/giorgio-agamben-a-question/ Original link: https://www.quodlibet.it/giorgio-agamben-una-domanda

Agamben, G. (2020b, May 2). *Medicine as a religion* (A. Kotsko, Trans.). https://itself.blog/2020/05/02/giorgio-agamben-medicine-as-religion/. Original link: https://www.quodlibet.it/giorgio-agamben-la-medicina-come-religione

Apuzzo, M., & Gebrekidan, S. (2021, January 29). Secret details seep out in deals governments have with drug makers. *New York Times*.

Bernholz, L. (2004). *Creating philanthropic capital markets: The deliberate evolution*. Wiley.

Bill Gates warns of epidemic that could kill over 30 million people. (2017, February 19). *Forbes*.

The birth of philanthrocapitalism. (2006, February 25). *The Economist*.

Bishop, M., & Green, M. (2009). *How the rich can save the world*. Bloomsbury Press.

Boutang, Y. M. (2011). *Cognitive capitalism*. Polity.

Braudel, F. (1977). *Afterthoughts on material civilization and capitalism* (P. Ranum, Trans.). Johns Hopkins University Press. (Original work published 1977)

Braudel, F. (1980). *On history* (S. Matthews, Trans.). University of Chicago Press. (Original work published 1969)

Braudel, F. (1996). *The Mediterranean and the Mediterranean world in the age of Philip II* (S. Reynolds, Trans.). University of California Press. (Original work published 1963)

Burns, R. (2019, April). New forms of philanthrocapitalism: Digital technologies and humanitarianism. *Antipode*, *51*(4), 1101–1122. https://doi.org/10.1111/anti.12534

Çakmakh, C., Demiralp, S., Kalemi-Özcan, Ş, Yeşiltaş, S., & Yildirim, M. (2021, January). *The economic case for global vaccinations: An epidemiological model with international production networks* (Working Paper 283395). National Bureau of Economic Research.

Chowdhury, A., & Jomo, K. S. (2020, May 26). Politics, profits undermine public interest in covid-19 vaccine race. Inter Press Service.

Chowdhury, A., & Jomo, K. S. (2021, July 13). Rich country hypocrisy exposed by vaccine inequalities. Inter Press Service.

Correa, C. M. (2021, July 19). Vaccination inequalities and the role of the multilateral system. Southviews No. 224. South Centre, pp. 1–2.

Cox, R. W. (1995). Civilizations: Encounters and transformations. *Studies in Political Economy*, *47*(1), 7–31. https://doi.org/10.1080/19187033.1995.11675358

Duke Global Health Institute. (2021). Retrieved January 30, from https://globalhealth.duke.edu/featured-publications/dghi-worldview

Fuchs, C. (2012). Towards Marxian internet studies. *TripleC: Cognition Communication co-Operation*, *10*(2), 392–412. https://doi.org/10.31269/triplec.v10i2.277

Hastings Center. (2020, March 16). Ethical framework for health care institutions & guidelines for institutional ethics services responding to the corona virus pandemic. https://www.thehastingscenter.org/ethicalframeworkcovid19/ 9

Heilleiner, E. (1997). Braudelian reflections on economic globalization: The historian as pioneer. In S. Gill & J. H. Mittelman (Eds.), *Innovation and transformation in international studies* (pp. 90–104). Cambridge University Press.

Mager, A. (2012). Algorithmic ideology: How capitalist ideology shapes search engines. *Information, Communication & Society*, *15*(1), 769–787. https://doi.org/10.1080/1369118X.2012.676056

McGoey, L. (2015). *No such thing as a free gift: The Gates Foundation and the price of philanthropy*. Verso.

Mueller, B., & Stevis-Gridneff, M. (2021, January 27). 'Solidarity is failing': EU: and Britain fight over vaccine doses. *New York Times.*

O'Neil, C. (2016). *Weapons of math destruction: How big data increases inequality and threatens democracy.* Crown Books.

Pasquale, F. (2015). *The black box society: The secret algorithms that control money and information.* Harvard University Press.

Peters, M., & Bulut, E. (Eds.). (2011). *Cognitive capitalism, education, and digital labor.* Peter Lang.

Piketty, T. (2020). *Capital and ideology.* Harvard University Press.

Reich, R. (2018). *Just giving: Why philanthropy is failing democracy and how it can be done better.* Princeton University Press.

Saker, L., Lee, B. C., Gilmore, A., & Campbell-Lendrum, D. H. (2004). *Globalization and infectious diseases: A review of the linkages.* World Health Organization. TDR/STR/SEB/ST/04.2.

Scholte, J. A. (2005). *Globalization: A critical introduction* (2nd ed., pp. 288–289). Palgrave Macmillan.

United Nations. (2021, June 7). WHO warns of 'two-track pandemic' as cases decline but vaccine inequity persists *UN News.*

Velásquez, G. (2020). *Re-thinking global and local manufacturing of medical products after COVID-19* (Research Paper 118). South Centre.

Vaccine nationalism: contested relationships between COVID-19 and globalization

Yanqiu Rachel Zhou

ABSTRACT

This article offers a review of the emergent literature on 'vaccine nationalism' - the act of gaining preferential access to newly developed vaccines by individual countries - in the context of COVID-19, paying close attention to the complex relationships between the global public health crisis and globalization. The coexistence of nationalist and globalist approaches to COVID-19 vaccines suggests simultaneous and contentious processes of globalization and deglobalization; the growing political and economic divide in the world; the lack of (or lag in) our consciousness of global interconnectedness, especially in non-economic spheres; and various structural barriers to global collaboration when facing a common threat to humanity's future. Although these tensions - not necessarily novel - are unlikely to end globalization given the extant intertwining of global economic networks, they have been sharpened and intensified during the pandemic and, thus, constitute a pivotal - or make-or-break - moment for us to critically imagine a postpandemic world.

Introduction

On 11 March 2020 the World Health Organization (WHO) declared the novel coronavirus (COVID-19) outbreak a global pandemic. The rapid spread of COVID-19 has also precipitated the unprecedentedly fast development of vaccines, something that heretofore has taken, on average, 10–15 years to accomplish (Rutschman, 2021a). Even months before any vaccine had been approved, however, high-income countries (HICs) that account for only a fraction of the global population had already ordered more than half of the projected early supply of doses. By mid-August 2020 the United States (US) had secured 800 million doses of at least 6 vaccines in development; the United Kingdom (UK) had purchased 340 million doses, with around 5 per capita; and the European Union (EU) and Japan had each ordered hundreds of millions of doses (Callaway, 2020). While the world's richest countries have reserved enough doses of the best vaccines to immunize their own populations multiple times (Bhutto, 2021), projected global manufacturing capacity also means limited and delayed access of low-income countries (LICs) to this important healthcare resource.

The present trend of 'vaccine nationalism' – the mindset and act of gaining preferential access to newly developed COVID-19 vaccines by individual countries (higher-income countries, in practice) – raises questions about nationalist approaches to the global public health crisis. After over four decades of the contemporary globalization processes, for instance, why is vaccine nationalism even possible despite increasing global economic integration and the development of global governance mechanisms? When 'we are only as strong as our weakest link' in a context of global pandemic, are those wealthy countries alone able to move themselves out of the crisis through their priority access to vaccines? What, moreover, does vaccine nationalism mean for a post-pandemic world, as well as for the future of globalization, when the significance of the nation-state as a world political entity has been both reinforced and challenged by the pandemic?

This article offers a review of the emergent literature on vaccine nationalism in the context of COVID-19, paying close attention to the complex relationships between COVID-19 and globalization. The first section presents some broad conditions that existed before the pandemic: in particular, US–China tensions and fragile global health governance in a context of frequent global health crises. These conditions also help to explain why COVID-19 vaccines, as well as the WHO, have become a new site of global competition and contestations during the pandemic. The second section focuses on the dynamics of vaccine nationalism, which should not be simplified as a sole product of domestic nationalism or a form of national crisis management strategy, but is, rather, a mix of geopolitics, international economic inequalities, global capitalism, and 'me-first' politics. The third section explores the COVID-19 Vaccines Global Access (COVAX) as a multilateral response to vaccine nationalism, emphasizing the challenges to and potentials of a globalist approach to equitable access to global public goods like vaccines. I contend that vaccine nationalism in the context of COVID-19 has exposed the dangers of nationalist responses to a simultaneous global emergency, and that it thus represents a pivotal moment in which the dynamics, courses, and directions of contemporary globalization processes must be critically reflected on and acted upon.

Contested globalization: changes to the 'world risk society' in the past decade or so

The 2007–2008 global financial crisis was a watershed moment in contemporary globalization processes on several levels (Garrett, 2010; Overholt, 2010). Empirically, the large-scale impacts of that crisis on the world economy have clearly brought what Ulrich Beck (1992, 1999) called 'risk society' – and, later, 'world risk society' – to higher-income countries, though risks have, arguably, have always been integral to lower-income countries' experiences of globalization. Modernity itself, according to Beck (1992, 1999), has created a world of uncontrollable risks (e.g. financial, ecological, and terrorism) and potential catastrophes, which neither respect state boundaries nor are clearly tied to one actor or source. The financial crisis signalled the risk inherent in global financial capitalism, and motivated massive post-crisis investments on both national and global levels to the purpose of mitigating future risks and preventing another, similar catastrophe (Sands, 2020). On a societal level, the fallout in many European nations from the global financial crisis, from unemployment and austerity measures to sovereign debt crises, has further complicated socio-economic inequalities and domestic politics (including nationalist sentiments and mobilization) (Polyakova & Fligstein, 2016; Wahl, 2017). In the EU countries most seriously hit (e.g. the UK, Italy, Ireland, France and Greece), Polyakova and Fligstein (2016) found that citizens' identification with the nation has grown dramatically, even as their identification with Europe has dwindled. The rise of nationalism in higher- and lower-income countries alike, climaxed in 2016 with Trump's election in the US and the UK's Brexit referendum. In these two countries the intersection of nationalism and anti-vaccine attitudes and movements is also apparent in the context of COVID-19, inhibiting their pursuit of 'herd immunity' despite the availability of vaccines (Foster & Feldman, 2021; Whitehead & Perry, 2020).

The impacts of the global financial crisis at a geopolitical level – in particular, US–China relations – are even more complex and far-reaching. In September 2008 China, which was largely immune to the blows inflicted by that crisis, surpassed Japan to become, at around $600 billion, the largest holder of US debt, and two years later became the world's second-largest economy (BBC, 2010; CFR, n.d.). In 2011 the US's trade deficit with China rose to an all-time high of $295.5 billion (CFR, n.d.). In its *World Development Report 2012*, the World Bank (2011) for the first time ranks China as an 'upper-middle-income country' (UMIC); only a decade before it was still a low-income nation. Seeing a rising China as its major competitor and a threat to its global hegemony, the US's policy on China has also changed. The tensions between the two countries were further exacerbated during the Trump Xi era, exemplified by their trade war before the COVID-19 pandemic and narrative battles during the pandemic (Jaworsky & Qiaoan, 2021; Yang, 2021). The worst moments of the latter include Trump calling COVID-19 'the Chinese virus', and a Chinese government spokesman promoting a conspiracy theory that the US Army brought the virus to Wuhan (Crowley et al., 2020).

As one of the major changes in global politics, the US–China rivalry has generated considerable uncertainty around – or, risks of – the future of the global economy, as well as global cooperation around COVID-19 responses (Esteves & van Staden, 2020). China's initial shutdown in the early period of the pandemic has revealed both the US's and higher-income countries' heavy reliance on that country for supplies – from personal protective equipment to components of pharmaceutical products – crucial to public health security (Evenett, 2020). In research and development (R&D), as well, the US and China account for almost half of the world's expenditure; they also collaborate more than any other two countries (Lee & Haupt, 2021). That collaboration was high during, for example, both the SARS (severe acute respiratory syndrome) and Ebola outbreaks, with China leading in SARS (SARS-CoV-1) publications and the US leading in Ebola publications (Sweileh, 2017). While collaboration between these two superpowers could enable timely global scientific responses to COVID-19 (SARS-CoV-2), the intensified geopolitical tensions are likely to endure, and be endured, beyond the current pandemic's resolution.

The past decade or so has, in fact, seen several global health crises. SARS, a pandemic caused by a coronavirus and that started in China in 2002, reached many countries, including higher-income ones like the US and Canada. One of the post-SARS responses at a global level is the WHO's adoption in the 2005 of the International Health Regulations (IHR), designed to keep the world informed about public health risks and events. It requires member states to have the ability to detect, assess, report, and respond to public health events, though in reality about two-thirds of countries lack that capacity (van Schaik et al., 2020). Implementing its IHR, the WHO has since declared six Public Health Emergencies of International Concern (PHEICs): the H1N1 influenza virus pandemic (2009), the resurgence of wild poliovirus (2014), the west Africa Ebola virus outbreak (2014), the Zika virus outbreak (2018), the Ebola outbreak in the Democratic Republic of the Congo (2019), and the current COVID-19 (2020) (Giesecke et al., 2019; Gordon, 2020). Despite these constantly emerging and reemerging infectious diseases, however, in its R&D Blueprint the WHO (2016) identified the problem of 'lack of R&D preparedness' for 'neglected diseases' like Ebola, a research area that is chronically unfunded. Although coronaviruses were listed as 'top emerging pathogens likely to cause severe outbreaks in the near future', to date there is no fully developed, tested, and approved SARS vaccine (Rutschman, 2021a; WHO, 2016, p. 22).

As a leading player in global health governance, furthermore, the WHO has been struggling with many challenges, including its own funding shortage, lack of enforcement power, lack of financial autonomy, the influence of geopolitics, and other organizations trespassing on its mandate, activities and, even, funding (Gostin, 2015; Hassan et al., 2021; Legge, 2020; van Schaik et al., 2020; Velasquez, 2020). The WHO's funding is a mix of mandatory assessed contributions (AC) from its member states (relative to the country's wealth and population) and voluntary contributions (VC) from donors (e.g. member states, philanthropic foundations, corporations, non-governmental organizations, and private individuals). While the WHO's operations costs have increased, member states' adherence to the zero-nominal growth policy for AC has restricted its budget growth and, in turn, increased its reliance on VC (Reddy et al., 2018). However, the steady rise of VC as a percentage of its overall budget, approaching 80% in 2014–2015, risks creating a situation where external donors dictate the WHO's priorities and action agenda (Clinton & Sridhar, 2017; Gostin, 2015). Until its withdrawal from the WHO during the pandemic, the US was its single biggest donor, contributing roughly 15% of its annual budget; it was followed by the Bill & Melinda Gates Foundation (BMGF), the UK, Germany, and Gavi, the Vaccine Alliance (GAVI) (Moulds, 2020). This structure may also help explain the WHO's volatile financial condition and why it has been a site of geopolitical contradictions between higher- and lower-income countries, as well as between the US and China (Clinton & Sridhar, 2017; Velasquez, 2020).

Characterized by acceleration in technology, economy, and social life (Rosa, 2013), contemporary globalization processes have also shaped the temporal dynamics of global pandemics and subsequent risks. While pathogens and viruses can travel as quickly as humans and cargo flow through global transportation networks, the quickening of global capitalist production processes has also sped up transmission between humans and other species, and subsequent virus mutations (Lee, 2003). By late December 2020, for example, nine countries – including The Netherlands, Denmark, the US, Spain, Italy, Lithuania, Sweden, Greece, and Canada – had reported outbreaks on mink farms (Schlanger, 2020). Subsequent COVID-19 mutations have generated worry about the possibility of the escape of the coronavirus into the wild mink population, and of the new variants' interference with the developed vaccines (Murray, 2020; WHO/Europe, 2020). Seeing SARS as a 'disease of speed', Zhou and Coleman (2016) pointed out that the potential global spread of the virus often 'accelerated' when it arrived at those highly ranked world cities – such as Hong Kong, Beijing, and Singapore – that are also hubs of global travel and economy. In 2004 Wuhan, the first epicentre of COVID-19 and China's seventh largest city, was not yet part of the world city networks, but by 2020 it had already become a beta world city, equivalent to Manchester, Geneva, and Lagos (GaWC, 2004, 2020).

Vaccine nationalism: a race against time and each other in an unequal world

Vaccine nationalism – 'the act of reserving millions of doses of new vaccines for domestic use during a transnational public health crisis' (Rutschman, 2021b, p. 9) – is viewed as a race 'among individual states to be the first on the market' (Jaworsky & Qiaoan, 2021, p. 298) and 'for priority rights to monopolize limited-production doses' (Daoudi, 2020, p. 2). It usually involves the use of advance market commitments or preproduction agreements between a national government and one or more pharmaceutical corporations engaged in late-stage development and production of leading vaccine candidates. Given that vaccine R&D is an area historically underinvested in because of its cost, risk, and time consumption, these advance commitments can function as incentives to attract private sector manufacturers that might otherwise choose to invest their time and resources in more profitable areas (Rutschman, 2021a, 2021b).

It is a far from novel or surprising phenomenon for rich countries to purchase vaccines and treatments years in advance. During the early stage of the 2009 H1N1 pandemic, for example, some wealthy countries (such as the US, Canada, and Australia) signed preproduction agreements with potential vaccine manufacturers – such as Sanofi, GlaxoSmithKline (GSK), and Novartis – to ensure their priority rights when the vaccines became available (Abbas, 2020). By early May 2009 it had been reported that the US had already placed advance orders that would enable it to buy over 600 million doses, though the projected global manufacturing capacity then was a best around 2 billion (Rutschman, 2021b). Upon the WHO's appeal, some wealthy countries pledged to donate 10% of their vaccine doses to poorer ones, but only when the worst of the pandemic had already passed and no further waves were expected (Abbas, 2020). The effects of vaccine nationalism, however, were never really put to the test, given the relatively fast wane of the H1N1 pandemic (Rutschman, 2021b). In fact, the glaring inequity of access to vaccines between wealthy and poor countries was already made apparent in 2006, when Indonesia upheld sharing its virus samples of H5N1 influenza with the WHO by citing 'viral sovereignty' (Hameiri, 2014; Fidler, 2012). Indonesia's worries about the unaffordability of vaccines developed by wealthy countries with lab and manufacturing capacity led to intriguing debates and negotiations on vaccine access and benefit sharing at the WHO level (Vezzani, 2010; Lange, 2012).

In the context of COVID-19 the dynamics of vaccine nationalism have been further complicated by changing US–China relations and the fact that both high-income economies (e.g. Italy, the USA, the UK, Australia, and Canada) and major emerging economies (e.g. China, South Africa, Brazil, and India) have all become epicentres over the course of the pandemic. As a result, COVID-19 vaccine R&D has been a fierce geopolitical race between powerful countries. In pursuing its 'America First' policy, the Trump administration quickly invested US $10 billion in several pharmaceutical corporations (e.g. Sanofi, GSK, AstraZeneca, Pfizer, Novavax, Moderna, and Johnson & Johnson) as vaccine candidates, either via direct financing or through vaccine procurement agreements, through its Operation Warp Speed (OWS) (Abbas, 2020; Daoudi, 2020). The latter is a public–private partnership initiated by the US government to facilitate and accelerate the development, manufacturing, and distribution of COVID-19 vaccines, therapeutics, and diagnostics.

The massive investment also means an unprecedented speed of vaccine R&D. By August 2020 the most promising Phase III vaccine candidates included those developed by AstraZeneca/Oxford (UK), Moderna (US), BioNTech (Germany) in collaboration with Pfizer (US) and Fosun Pharma (China), the last of which was later reduced to the status of a distributor (Wong, 2021). On 9 November 2020 Pfizer and BioNTech declared through a press release – not through peer-reviewed publications, though – that their COVID-19 vaccine (i.e. BNT162b2) had an effective prevention rate of more than 90% (Badrinath, 2021; Pfizer, 2020). By the end of 2020 Russia had approved its vaccine, named 'Sputnik V' in tribute to the Soviet Union's triumphal first artificial space satellite in 1957, during the Cold War; China was conducting final trials of its five vaccine candidates; and the US had approved the vaccines from Pfizer and Moderna (BBC, 2020; Choi, 2021; Wong, 2021). While rich countries, with 14% of the world's population, have stockpiled 53% of the best vaccines (i.e. those with the highest efficacy) – all Moderna vaccines and almost all of the Pfizer/BioNTech vaccines will go to them – only 25 vaccine doses had been administered in the whole of sub-Saharan Africa as of the last week of January 2021 (Bhutto, 2021).

Vaccine nationalism, producing extremely inequitable vaccine access, both illustrates and reinforces the long-standing inequalities in public health between higher- and lower-income countries. Without timely access to vaccines for health workers and high-risk populations, lower-income countries – generally densely populated, with weak health systems and higher disease burdens – will experience a vicious circle of widespread transmission, the collapse of healthcare systems, and humanitarian crises, which will continue to threaten the entire global population and prolong the pandemic (Abbas, 2020; Daoudi, 2021; WHO, 2021a). In addition, vaccine nationalism, part of the broader vaccine race permeated with the bloc logic of the Cold War, has also sundered the world into two distinct groups (Daoudi, 2021). While vaccine nationalism has attracted participation from higher-income countries, many lower-income ones have aligned with China's 'vaccine diplomacy' (Daoudi, 2021; Gruszczynski & Wu, 2021; Karásková & Blablová, 2021). After President Xi's vow in May 2020 to make Chinese COVID-19 vaccines 'a global public good' to ensure 'vaccine accessibility and affordability in developing countries', in June 2021 China also launched, jointly with 28 other countries (e.g. Afghanistan, Bangladesh, Chile, Colombia, Indonesia, Saudi Arabia, United Arab Emirates, and Uzbekistan) its 'Initiative for Belt and Road Partnership on COVID-19 Vaccines Cooperation' (Ministry of Foreign Affairs, 2021; A. Wang, 2021; Weaton, 2020). Yet this gulf continues to widen, not only undermining the transnational solidarity required to tackle COVID-19 as a global problem, but also deepening the conflict with the logic of global health that supports international collaboration over immediate nation-state interests (Lee & Haupt, 2021). Making COVID-19 a zero-sum geopolitical power game, with winners and losers, will heighten tensions between the immunized and the nonimmunized, between inequality and security, and between globalism and nationalism, eventually resulting in 'a race to the bottom' where there can be no true winner (Choi, 2021; Daoudi, 2020; Wong, 2021).

As well, vaccine nationalism reveals the mutually reinforcing relationship between protectionism, populism, authoritarianism, and racism/xenophobia (Z. Wang, 2021). Pursuing vaccine nationalism means indifference to others, or an 'almost total absence of political feeling for the world' on the one hand, and a 'short-sighted, potentially risky, morally indefensible, and practically inefficient' approach to global contagion on the other hand (Abbas, 2020, p. 2; James & Valluvan, 2020, p. 1245). Emphasizing COVID-19 as an exogenous danger to national security, vaccine nationalism risks exacerbating domestic nationalism and constructing the 'other' (e.g. certain ethnic groups) within national borders (Jaworsky & Qiaoan, 2021; Z. Wang, 2021). In the UK, for example, vaccine nationalism has been exaggerated and distorted, by a largely Eurosceptic press, into a Brexit-related issue (Hearne, 2021). When national states become the primary decision makers about global health emergency responses (e.g. vaccine access and border control) during a pandemic, the power of the nation-state as a fundamental organizing unit of global politics, as well as the pre-existing trends away from globalization, have *de facto* strengthened (Esteves & van Staden, 2020). For a global problem like COVID-19, nevertheless, a 'me-first approach [is] self-defeating', because no country can solve it alone (WHO, 2021a).

Furthermore, vaccine nationalism as a global phenomenon represents a nationalist turn that undercuts multilateral and collective approaches to global problems. Exhausting the early vaccine supply, vaccine nationalism has directly challenged the United Nations' Sustainable Development Goals (SDGs) when it comes to equitable and fair access to vaccines for all, as well as the WHO's COVAX initiative, which is designed to get vaccines to low- and middle-income countries (LMICs) (Nhamo et al., 2020; The Guardian, 2021). The dilemma is also compounded by the fact that 'most manufacturers have prioritized regulatory approval in rich countries where the profits are highest, rather than submitting full dossiers to WHO' (WHO, 2021a). In this sense, vaccine nationalism – fuelled by contractual bilateralism – has further weakened the authority of the WHO and, in turn, the multilateral systems of global health governance. Seeing vaccine nationalism or any other 'nationalistic approach to the allocation of health goods needed transnationally' as an extension of competition-driven frameworks in the pharmaceutical industry, Rutschman (2021b) further advocates our critical reflection on the 'systemically siloed approach' to vaccine R&D, which regards health goods more as profitable commodities than as global public goods, and is integral to 'the wobbly post–World War II institutional architecture of global health' (p. 13 and p. 14).

COVAX: a globalist but temporary accelerator

Co-led by the WHO, GAVI, and the Coalition for Epidemic Preparedness Innovations (CEPI), the COVAX facility was launched in June 2020, the same month the US officially withdrew from the WHO. Aiming to ensure the worldwide vaccination of the most vulnerable populations and healthcare workers with approximately two billion doses by the end of 2021, this new multilateral procurement mechanism reflects an attempt at a global level to mitigate the effects of vaccine nationalism and grant access to countries who do not have the fiscal or political means to secure bilateral agreements with vaccine manufacturers (Eccleston-Turner & Upton, 2021; Gemünden & Thiel, 2021; Sharma et al., 2021). COVAX is the vaccine pillar of the Access to COVID-19 Tools Accelerator (ACT-A), 'a global and *time-limited* collaboration' launched by the WHO and partners in early 2020 to accelerate the development and production of, and equitable global access to, new COVID-19 essential health technologies (WHO, 2020a; Italic added). The three co-leaders play a separate but supplementary role in this platform: the WHO oversees 'policy and allocation' issues, CEPI coordinates vaccine 'development and manufacturing', and GAVI is responsible for 'procurement and delivery at-scale' (cited in Rutschman, 2021a, p. 194).

Both CEPI and GAVI are public–private partnerships. As the first large-scale product development partnership focusing solely on vaccines, CEPI was launched in 2017 in the aftermath of the 2014–2016 Ebola outbreak; its funders include over two dozen countries, the BMGF, the Wellcome Trust in the UK, and the European Commission (CEPI, n.d.; European Commission, 2020). Only two weeks after essential genomic information about the novel coronavirus was first made available to the scientific community, in January 2020 did it start three funding programmes to accelerate the development of vaccine candidates (CEPI, 2020; Rutschman, 2021a). Created in 2000, Switzerland-based GAVI focuses exclusively on vaccine supply and procurement and in the past 2 decades has introduced 496 vaccines and contributed to the vaccination of 760 million children around the world (Rutschman, 2021a; UNICEF, 2021). Setting up the process of 'what might become the largest vaccine procurement scheme in history', COVAX's quick actions are attributable to CEPI and GAVI's pre-exiting relationships with key players (e.g. donors, manufacturers, and NGOs) and established global networks (e.g. for freight, logistics and storage), as well as to UNICEF's – that is, its key delivery partner's – longstanding expertise in procurement and logistics (Rutschman, 2021a, p. 191; UNICEF, 2021). While GAVI, like the BMGF, emerges as a new (that is, not traditional) and increasingly powerful player in the field of global health governance, it also represents a controversial trend in the field. The shift to the private–public partnership model also means a move towards narrower mandates, problem-focused initiatives (including funding), and/or technical solutions, and away from broader systemic goals of global health (Clinton & Sridhar, 2017; Storeng, 2014).

Unlike other WHO initiatives targeting LMICs, COVAX urges the participation of HICs in this global project. While the platform represents the 'best hope' for LMICs to access vaccines, the WHO also highlights its importance as a risk 'diversification' and 'insurance' system for wealthy countries that have pursued bilateral advanced agreements with vaccine manufacturers (Gavi, 2020; WHO, 2020b). By pooling resources and offering larger orders of vaccines, COVAX also means an opportunity to negotiate lower prices on behalf of the participating countries. Despite 'an unprecedented mobilization of sovereign funders and private sector, philanthropic and multilateral contributors', however, by May 2021 the ACT-A still faced a funding gap of 19 billion US dollars (including 2.6 billion for vaccines), and will need a further 35–45 billion dollars next year to vaccinate most adults around the world (WHO, 2021b). Meanwhile, the uneven participation of some powerful players is hard to ignore. In September 2020, only three months after its launch, the EU joined COVAX, and China did so the following month (Reuters, 2021). It was not until February 2021, however, that the Biden administration promised to join (Baker, 2021). The apparent hesitancy may reflect geopolitical relationships among these countries and regions and their reservations about relying on the facility for faster vaccine access. Take the EU when COVID-19 arrived: on one hand, its quick action in filling the vacuum – both financially and politically – created by the US's withdrawal marks a shift in its approach to the WHO as a multilateral organization for global health; on the other hand, its support for the WHO – or, the global response to COVID-19 through multilateral platforms – was accompanied by an initial decision not to engage with COVAX and its aggressive pursuit of bilateral agreements with vaccine manufacturers (European Commission, 2020; van Schaik et al., 2020). This 'half-in, half-out approach to multilateral cooperation', however, may reinforce fears about COVAX's inability to access vaccines before HICs, and thus be detrimental to the facility in the long term (Eccleston-Turner & Upton, 2021, p. 14).

Participating countries are divided into 2: (a) 'self-financing' HICs and UMICs, which make upfront payments to support vaccine development; and (b) 92 MICs and LICs, which are funded through COVAX's Advanced Market Commitment (AMC), which is a financing mechanism to raise funds, mostly official development assistance (ODA), to pay for their vaccine supply (Emanuel et al., 2021; McAdams et al., 2020). The facility uses a two-phase allocation mechanism. In phase 1, countries receive vaccine doses in equal proportion, to cover up to 20% of their total population, with an interim target of 3%. After phase 1 is completed, in phase 2 the proportional approach will be replaced by a targeted distribution based on a country's needs (e.g. vulnerabilities, disease burden, and health system capacity) (Emanuel et al., 2021; Sharma et al., 2021). Once self-financing countries receive doses of vaccine to cover 20% of their population, they will be free to distribute domestically according to their own priorities. Yet the same requirement does not apply to the funded countries, impairing their ability to pursue multiple vaccine purchase or pre-purchase pathways. As well, current COVAX policies recommend, but do not require, self-funded countries to donate vaccines if they have extra (Rutschman, 2021a, 2021b). In other words, HICs have more flexibility when it comes to where they can access vaccines and how they can use them.

The distinction between countries based on economic purchasing power suggests 'skewed prioritization of financial metrics over global public health', and risks further separating the higher-income countries from the lower-income ones; both developments are unconducive to a global equitable distribution framework (Rutschman, 2021a, pp. 197–198, 2021b). Although the proportional allocation may help incentivize wealthy countries to participate in COVAX (given their importance for its financing), it is morally problematic not to take a country's need into account from the start and not to prioritize the most vulnerable or worst off (Emanuel et al., 2021; Sharma et al., 2021). Furthermore, the COVAX's vaccine allocation schemes seem to be based on the responses of nation-states instead of the interests of global citizenry, though in ethics the unit of concern for justice is individuals, not countries (Emanuel et al., 2021). Israel, a participant in the COVAX facility, and a country with one of the highest COVID-19 vaccination rates in the world, for example, initially denied responsibility for vaccinating the Palestinians of the Occupied Territories (Dyer, 2021). In the context of the 'One China policy', Taiwan has also found it challenging to secure COVID-19 vaccines through either participation in COVAX or purchase from pharmaceutical corporations (e.g. Pfizer/BioNTech) (Zhong & Schuetze, 2021). Despite accelerated development of COVID-19 vaccines, moreover, Eccleston-Turner and Upton (2021) argue that lower-income countries' access to the benefit will be limited. In addition to vaccine nationalism, another significant barrier faced by most lower-income countries is the lack of infrastructure (e.g. for transportation, storage, and manufacturing) to actualize the global allocation mechanism, something else that was revealed during the H1N1 pandemic (Daoudi, 2020; Eccleston-Turner & Upton, 2021).

It is worth noting that in October 2020 India and South Africa requested the World Trade Organization (WTO) to temporarily suspend intellectual property (IP) rights so that COVID-19 vaccines and other new technologies could be accessible to lower-income countries for the duration of the pandemic (MSF, 2020; Usher, 2020). That proposal, though, was rejected by HICs (e.g. the UK, the USA, Canada, Norway, and the EU), which argue that the IP system is required to incentivize new inventions of vaccines, diagnostics, and treatments, and that equitable vaccine access can be achieved through other mechanisms, such as the donor-funded COVAX (Usher, 2020). In May 2020 India and South Africa revised their proposal for the patent waiver on COVID-19 vaccines in light of the devastating second wave of the pandemic (caused by the Delta variant) in India, and has since gained increasing support from heterogeneous actors, including the BRICS countries (Brazil, Russia, India, China, and South Africa), more lower-incomes countries (e.g. in Latin America), local and international civil society organizations, and, surprisingly, the US and the EU (CCPA, 2021; Contreras, 2021; Deutsche Welle, 2021; Economic Times, 2021; Laskar, 2021; MSF, 2020; Sibal, 2021). Yet an IP waiver alone will not solve the COVID-19 vaccine access challenge because of the time ramping up manufacturing will take and lower-income countries' constrained capacity (e.g. infrastructure, technology, and know-how) to mass produce pharmaceutical products (Daoudi, 2020; Gonsalves & Yamey, 2021). Nevertheless, it is yet to be seen whether and how the contestations around the IP rights of COVID-19 vaccines will enable new opportunities of global health advocacy and cross-border social solidarity under the stress of the pandemic, especially considering the earlier tremendous success of AIDS treatment activism at the WTO 'despite careful opposition from powerful transnational corporate firms and their home governments' (Odell & Sell, 2006, p. 85). While COVAX cannot and should not operate as a stand-alone programme to address the problems of COVID-19 vaccine access, such examples of transnational activism remind us of the importance of other, less visible, players, such as lower-income countries themselves, as well as the pharmaceutical industry and NGOs, in facilitating equitable vaccine access.

Although COVAX is an important and timely step toward global equitable access to COVID-19 vaccines, its other challenges and limitations should not be overlooked. Despite the participation of multiple actors, their bargaining asymmetries in this global health partnership – especially between players on opposite sides of the public–private divide – are clear (Rutschman, 2021a). Heavily favouring pharmaceutical corporations, the funding mechanism of COVAX provides them with a win-win situation, and an opportunity to benefit regardless of whether their vaccine candidate ever goes on to gain regulatory approval (Eccleston-Turner & Upton, 2021). The opacity of the conditions (e.g. pricing, patent protection, and sanctions) has been noted in the contracts between pharmaceutical corporations and CEPI, as well as in wealthy countries that have engaged in vaccine nationalism (Abbas, 2020; Dyer, 2021; Usher, 2021). The COVAX's reliance on philanthropic funding for financing also suggests its financial vulnerability to donor fatigue (Rutschman, 2021a). The proliferation of public–private partnerships – as in both COVAX and vaccine nationalism, as well as in global health governance architecture – again demonstrates that private solutions and interests (or market mechanisms) are generally privileged over public approaches, and constitutes a further deepening of the neoliberal management of global health crises (Ruckert & Labonté, 2014; Rutschman, 2021a). While a two-tier system (i.e. multilateral vaccine governance and vaccine nationalism) is likely to endure, COVAX should consider working with (by pushing and rewarding, for example) wealthy countries in developing good bilateral deals with vaccine manufactures that can benefit LICs (McAdams et al., 2020). As well, the temporary nature of COVAX means a lack of permanent structures or long-term solutions to a recurring problem at a supranational level (Rutschman, 2021a). Consolidating and institutionalizing COVAX as a multilateral platform beyond this pandemic is, however, in the health, economic, and security interests of higher-income countries, and will also limit the space for vaccine diplomacy as currently conducted by China, Russia, and the US (Gemünden & Thiel, 2021).

Conclusion

Pandemics like COVID-19 are not merely about an undesirable outcome of contemporary globalization processes; they also chart the course and shape the future of globalization by, for example, creating new sites and connections of global contestation. Indeed,

> the global does not consist merely of a series of flows floating above or between national spaces or sets of interconnected sites, but rather refers to emergent problems […] that unevenly permeate relations on a planetary scale, producing shared predicaments in spite of empirical differences. (Rudnyckyj & Whitington, 2020, p. 1043)

While thanks to vaccination re-opening has become a tangible reality in wealthy countries like the UK, the US, and Canada, we are simultaneously witnessing the COVID-19 catastrophe in India, which is the home of the world's largest vaccine manufacturer, the Serum Institute of India (under licence from AstraZeneca), but which nevertheless is itself experiencing a major internal shortage (Ellyatt, 2021). While Pfizer is currently seeking approval from wealthy countries for a third vaccine booster shot, only 20% of people in LMICs will be fully vaccinated by the end of 2021 *even if* COVAX reaches its targets (Cheng, 2021). In a globalized world afflicted with geo-economic inequalities, nation-states' varying capacities to respond in a *timely* way to the *simultaneity* of a global health crisis have constituted and reinforced the crisis itself (Zhou & Coleman, 2016). Although the unprecedentedly speedy vaccine development is viewed as key to mitigating the effects of COVID-19 and moving toward a post-pandemic world, a more important question is whether all countries are able to share the benefit of that speed, and whether some may be even forced to decelerate. In the contexts of a highly integrated world economy and relatively slower vaccine rollout in many LMICs countries, how long can wealthy countries sustain, by themselves, their temporal advantages to accelerate and to maintain health?

This article reveals the contested relationships between COVID-19 and globalization. First, although vaccine nationalism reflects some wealthy countries' desire to accelerate their movement toward a post-pandemic world, the lack of timely access to vaccines in many lower-income countries may, rather, prolong COVID-19's threat (including its mutations) across the globe. Second, while COVAX as a timely but temporary accelerator at a supranational level is now presented as a hope for lower-income countries to access COVID-19 vaccines, vaccine nationalism has fundamentally challenged the status of multilateralism as one of the pillars of contemporary globalization processes. Third, the geopolitics of vaccine nationalism must be understood in the context of increasingly intense US–China relations (including their vaccine race and diplomacy), which have further exacerbated the complexities and uncertainties surrounding the future of globalization. Fourth, short-term nationalist responses to the global pandemic may also enable the re-naturalization of the nation-state (by resorting to it for responding to a global crisis), which could, in the long run, compromise collective capacities to tackle other impending global crises, such as other pandemics and climate disasters.

Although these tensions – not necessarily novel – are unlikely to end globalization given the extant intertwining of global economic networks, they have been sharpened and intensified during the pandemic and, thus, constitute a pivotal – or make-or-break – moment for us to critically imagine a post-pandemic world. The coexistence of nationalist and globalist approaches to COVID-19 vaccines suggests simultaneous and contentious processes of globalization and deglobalization; the growing political and economic divide in the world; the lack of (or lag in) our consciousness of global interconnectedness, especially in non-economic spheres; and various structural barriers to global collaboration when facing a common threat to humanity's future. In this sense, exploring vaccine nationalism as a problem that cuts across multiple sites of globalization – in terms of geopolitics, technocentrism, institutional spheres, global consciousness, sense of hierarchy, and time–space relations, for example – sheds light on the contentious politics of this global health crisis and, in turn, opens up theoretical perspectives and discursive spaces for understandings of globalization processes, in which both multifaceted inequalities and transplanetary solidarity have become unprecedentedly sophisticated and urgent.

Acknowledgements

I wish to express my appreciation to the editors of this special issue – Drs Kevin Gray and Barry Gills – for this opportunity and for their guidance and to anonymous reviewers of this journal for their insightful comments on the article. I also thank Kristy Yiu for her research assistance at the early stage of this project.

Disclosure statement

No potential conflict of interest was reported by the author.

Funding

This work was supported by the Social Sciences and Humanities Research Council of Canada (SSHRCC) [grant number 435-2020-0139].

References

Abbas, M. Z. (2020). *Practical implications of 'vaccine nationalism': A short-sighted and risky approach in response to COVID-19* (South Centre, Research Paper, 124). https://eprints.qut.edu.au/206694/1/73000748.pdf

Badrinath, P. (2021). Money, market, media, and vaccine nationalism in the pandemic era. *BMJ, 372*, n630. https://doi.org/10.1136/bmj.n630

Baker, S. (2021, February 2). The US is finally joining the push for global vaccine access. *Business Insider.* https://www.businessinsider.com/us-joins-covax-experts-say-wont-help-poorer-nations-much-2021-1

BBC. (2010, February 14). China overtakes Japan as world's second-biggest economy. https://www.bbc.com/news/business-12427321#:~:text=China%20has%20overtaken%20Japan%20as,trillion%20in%20the%20same%20period

BBC. (2020, December 19). Covid: US approves Moderna as second vaccine. https://www.bbc.com/news/world-us-canada-55370999

Beck, U. (1992). *Risk society: Towards a new modernity.* Sage.

Beck, U. (1999). *World risk society.* Polity Press.

Bhutto, F. (2021, April 4). The world's richest countries are hoarding vaccines. This is morally indefensible. *The Guardian.* https://www.theguardian.com/commentisfree/2021/mar/17/rich-countries-hoarding-vaccines-us-eu-africa

Callaway, E. (2020, August 24). The unequal scramble for coronavirus vaccines – By numbers. *Nature.* https://www.nature.com/articles/d41586-020-02450-x

Canadian Centre for Policy Alternatives (CCPA). (2021, May 23). *Civil society letter supporting India's and South Africa's proposal for a TRIPS agreement waiver for COVID-19 treatments.* https://www.policyalternatives.ca/newsroom/updates/civil-society-letter-supporting-indias-and-south-africas-proposal-trips-agreement

CEPI. (2020, January 23). CEPI to fund three programmes to develop vaccines against the novel coronavirus, nCoV-2019. https://cepi.net/news_cepi/cepi-to-fund-three-programmes-to-develop-vaccines-against-the-novel-coronavirus-ncov-2019/

CEPI. (n.d.). *Who we are.* https://cepi.net/about/whoweare/

Cheng, M. (2021, July 12). WHO: Rich countries should donate vaccines, not use boosters. *Associated Press.* https://apnews.com/article/europe-business-health-government-and-politics-coronavirus-pandemic-02b1157d4f0def0460c9c4548f1c7679

Choi, S. H. (2021). *How the pandemic undermined US hegemony in Asia-Pacific: The COVID-19 vaccine war and the south China sea.* Atlas Institute for International Affairs. https://www.internationalaffairshouse.org/how-the-pandemic-undermined-us-hegemony-in-asia-pacific-the-covid-19-vaccine-war-and-the-south-china-sea/

Clinton, C., & Sridhar, D. (2017). Who pays for cooperation in global health? A comparative analysis of WHO, the World Bank, the global fund to fight HIV/AIDS, tuberculosis and malaria, and Gavi, the vaccine alliance. *The Lancet, 390*(10091), 324–332. https://doi.org/10.1016/S0140-6736(16)32402-3

Contreras, J. L. (2021). US support for a WTO waiver of COVID-19 intellectual property. *Intereconomics, 56*(3), 179–180. https://doi.org/10.1007/s10272-021-0976-7

Council for Foreign Relations (CFR). (n.d.). *U.S. relations with China: 1949–2021.* https://www.cfr.org/timeline/us-relations-china

Crowley, M., Wong, E., & Jakes, L. (2020, March 22). Coronavirus drives the U.S. and China deeper into global power struggle. *New York Times.* https://www.nytimes.com/2020/03/22/us/politics/coronavirus-us-china.html

Daoudi, S. (2020). *Vaccine nationalism in the context of COVID-19: An obstacle to the containment of the pandemic.* Policy Center for the New South. https://media.africaportal.org/documents/PB_-_20-71_Salma_Daoudi_EN.pdf

Deutsche Welle. (2021, June 28). India, South Africa bid to ban COVID vaccine patents finds few takers in Latin America. https://www.dw.com/en/india-south-africa-bid-to-ban-covid-vaccine-patents-finds-few-takers-in-latin-america/a-58048258

Doctors Without Borders/Médecins Sans Frontières (MSF). (2020, October 7). Governments make request to WTO for intellectual property waiver for all countries until herd immunity is reached. https://www.doctorswithoutborders.org/what-we-do/news-stories/news/india-and-south-africa-propose-no-patents-covid-19-medicines-and-tools

Dyer, O. (2021). Covid-19: Countries are learning what others paid for vaccines. *BMJ, 372*, n281. https://doi.org/10.1136/bmj.n281

Eccleston-Turner, M. A. R. K., & Upton, H. (2021). International collaboration to ensure equitable access to vaccines for COVID-19: The ACT-accelerator and the COVAX facility. *The Milbank Quarterly, 99*(2), 426–449. https://doi.org/10.1111/1468-0009.12503

Economic Times. (2021, June 1). BRICS backs India-South Africa's COVID-19 vaccine patent waiver proposal. https://economictimes.indiatimes.com/news/india/brics-backs-india-south-africas-covid-19-vaccine-patent-waiver-proposal/articleshow/83149877.cms?from=mdr

Ellyatt, H. (2021, May 5). India is the home of the world's biggest producer of Covid vaccines. But it's facing a major internal shortage. *CNBC.* https://www.cnbc.com/2021/05/05/why-covid-vaccine-producer-india-faces-major-shortage-of-doses.html

Emanuel, E. J., Luna, F., Schaefer, G. O., Tan, K. C., & Wolff, J. (2021). Enhancing the WHO's proposed framework for distributing COVID-19 vaccines among countries. *American Journal of Public Health, 111*(3), 371–373. https://doi.org/10.2105/AJPH.2020.306098

Esteves, P., & van Staden, C. (2020). *Policy insights: US and Chinese COVID-19 health outreach to Africa and Latin America: A comparison.* South African Institute of International Affairs. https://media.africaportal.org/documents/Policy-Insights-98-esteves-van-staden.pdf

European Commission. (2020). *Global cooperation.* https://ec.europa.eu/info/research-and-innovation/research-area/health-research-and-innovation/coronavirus-research-and-innovation/global-cooperation_en

Evenett, S. J. (2020). Chinese whispers: COVID-19, global supply chains in essential goods, and public policy. *Journal of International Business Policy, 3*(4), 408–429. https://doi.org/10.1057/s42214-020-00075-5

Fidler, D. P. (2012). Negotiating equitable access to influenza vaccines: Global health diplomacy and the controversies surrounding avian influenza H5N1 and pandemic influenza H1N1. In E. Rosskam & I. Kickbusch (Eds.), *Negotiating and navigating global health: Case studies in global health diplomacy* (pp. 161–172). World Scientific.

Foster, R., & Feldman, M. (2021). From 'Brexhaustion' to 'Covidiots': The United Kingdom and the populist future. *Journal of Contemporary European Research, 17*(2), 116–127. https://doi.org/10.30950/jcer.v17i2.1231

Garrett, G. (2010). G2 in G20: China, the United States and the world after the global financial crisis. *Global Policy, 1*(1), 29–39. https://doi.org/10.1111/j.1758-5899.2009.00014.x

Gavi. (2020, September 3). COVAX explained. https://www.gavi.org/vaccineswork/covax-explained

Gemünden, M., & Thiel, J. (2021). COVAX needs a political future. *Policy Perspectives, 9/4.* https://css.ethz.ch/content/dam/ethz/special-interest/gess/cis/center-for-securities-studies/pdfs/PP9-4_2021-EN.pdf

Giesecke, J., Bedford, J., Enria, D., Heymann, D. L., Ihekweazu, C., Kobinger, G., Lane, C., Memish, Z., Oh, M.-d., Sall, A., Schuchat, A., Ungchusak, K., & Wieler, L. (2019). The truth about PHEICs. *The Lancet.* Advance online publication. https://doi.org/10.1016/S0140-6736(19)31566-1

Globalization and World Cities Research Network (GaWc). (2004). *The world according to GaWC 2004.* https://www.lboro.ac.uk/gawc/world2004t.html

Globalization and World Cities Research Network (GaWC). (2020). *The world according to GaWC 2020.* https://www.lboro.ac.uk/gawc/world2020t.html

Gonsalves, G., & Yamey, G. (2021). The covid-19 vaccine patent waiver: A crucial step towards a "people's vaccine". *BMJ, 373,* n1249. https://doi.org/10.1136/bmj.n1249

Gordon, A. (2020). WHO declares global health emergency over coronavirus: 4 questions answered. *The Conversation.* https://theconversation.com/who-declares-global-health-emergency-over-coronavirus-4-questions-answered-130940

Gostin, L. O. (2015). The future of the World Health Organization: Lessons learned from Ebola. *Milbank Quarterly, 93*(3), 475. https://doi.org/10.1111/1468-0009.12134

Gruszczynski, L., & Wu, C.-H. (2021). Between the high ideals and reality: Managing COVID-19 vaccine nationalism. *European Journal of Risk Regulation.* Advance online publication. https://doi.org/10.1017/err.2021.9

Hameiri, S. (2014). Avian influenza, 'viral sovereignty', and the politics of health security in Indonesia. *The Pacific Review, 27*(3), 333–356. https://doi.org/10.1080/09512748.2014.909523

Hassan, I., Mukaigawara, M., King, L., Fernandes, G., & Sridhar, D. (2021). Hindsight is 2020? Lessons in global health governance one year into the pandemic. *Nature Medicine, 27*(3), 396–400. https://doi.org/10.1038/s41591-021-01272-2

Hearne, D. (2021). *Vaccine nationalism.* Centre for Brexit Studies Blog, Centre for Brexit Studies. http://www.open-access.bcu.ac.uk/id/eprint/11469

James, M., & Valluvan, S. (2020). Coronavirus conjuncture: Nationalism and pandemic states. *Sociology, 54* (6), 1238–1250. https://doi.org/10.1177/0038038520969114

Jaworsky, B. N., & Qiaoan, R. (2021). The politics of blaming: The narrative battle between China and the US over COVID-19. *Journal of Chinese Political Science, 26*, 295–315. https://doi.org/10.1007/s11366-020-09690-8

Karásková, I., & Blablová, V. (2021, March 24). The logic of China's vaccine diplomacy. *The Diplomat.* https://thediplomat.com/2021/03/the-logic-of-chinas-vaccine-diplomacy/

Lange, J. E. (2012). Negotiating issues related to pandemic influenza preparedness: The sharing of influenza viruses and access to vaccines and other benefits. In E. Rosskam & I. Kickbusch (Eds.), *Negotiating and navigating global health: Case studies in global health diplomacy* (pp. 129–159). World Scientific.

Laskar, R. H. (2021, May 1). India, South Africa to make fresh push for waiver of vaccine patents at WTO. https://www.hindustantimes.com/india-news/india-south-africa-to-make-fresh-push-for-waiver-of-vaccine-patents-at-wto-101619886294125.html

Lee, J. J., & Haupt, J. P. (2021). Scientific collaboration on COVID-19 amidst geopolitical tensions between the US and China. *The Journal of Higher Education, 92*(2), 303–329. https://doi.org/10.1080/00221546.2020.1827924

Lee, K. (2003). *Globalization and health: An introduction.* Palgrave Macmillan.

Legge, D. G. (2020). COVID-19 response exposes deep flaws in global health governance. *Global Social Policy, 20*(3), 383–387. https://doi.org/10.1177/1468018120966659

McAdams, D., McDade, K. K., Ogbuoji, O., Johnson, M., Dixit, S., & Yamey, G. (2020). Incentivising wealthy nations to participate in the COVID-19 vaccine global access facility (COVAX): A game theory perspective. *BMJ Global Health, 5*(11), e003627. https://doi.org/10.1136/bmjgh-2020-003627

Ministry of Foreign Affairs, People's Republic of China. (2021, June 24). Initiative for belt and road partnership on COVID-19 vaccines cooperation. https://www.fmprc.gov.cn/mfa_eng/wjdt_665385/2649_665393/t1886387.shtml

Moulds, J. (2020). How is the World Health Organization funded? *World Economic Forum.* https://www.weforum.org/agenda/2020/04/who-funds-world-health-organization-un-coronavirus-pandemic-covid-trump/

Murray, A. (2020, November 11). Coronavirus: Denmark shaken by cull of millions of mink. *BBC.* https://www.bbc.com/news/world-europe-54890229

Nhamo, G., Chikodzi, D., Kunene, H. P., & Mashula, N. (2020). COVID-19 vaccines and treatments nationalism: Challenges for low-income countries and the attainment of the SDGs. *Global Public Health, 16*(3), 319–339. https://doi.org/10.1080/17441692.2020.1860249

Odell, J. S., & Sell, S. (2006). Reframing the issue: The WTO coalition on intellectual property and public health, 2001. In J. S. Odell (ed.), *Negotiating trade: Developing countries in the WTO and NAFTA* (pp. 85–114). Cambridge: Cambridge University Press.

Overholt, W. H. (2010). China in the global financial crisis: Rising influence, rising challenges. *The Washington Quarterly, 33*(1), 21–34. https://doi.org/10.1080/01636600903418652

Pfizer. (2020, November 9). Pfizer and BioNTech announce vaccine candidate against COVID-19 achieved success in first interim analysis from Phase 3 study. https://www.pfizer.com/news/press-release/press-release-detail/pfizer-and-biontech-announce-vaccine-candidate-against

Polyakova, A., & Fligstein, N. (2016). Is European integration causing Europe to become more nationalist? Evidence from the 2007–9 financial crisis. *Journal of European Public Policy, 23*(1), 60–83. https://doi.org/10.1080/13501763.2015.1080286

Reddy, S. K., Mazhar, S., & Lencucha, R. (2018). The financial sustainability of the World Health Organization and the political economy of global health governance: A review of funding proposals. *Globalization and Health, 14*(1), 1–11. https://doi.org/10.1186/s12992-018-0436-8

Reuters. (2021, April 21). A year in the COVID-19 vaccine scheme COVAX. https://www.reuters.com/business/healthcare-pharmaceuticals/year-covid-19-vaccine-scheme-covax-2021-04-21/

Rosa, H. (2013). *Social acceleration: A new theory of modernity.* Columbia University Press.

Ruckert, A., & Labonté, R. (2014). Public–private partnerships (PPPs) in global health: The good, the bad and the ugly. *Third World Quarterly, 35*(9), 1598–1614. https://doi.org/10.1080/01436597.2014.970870

Rudnyckyj, D., & Whitington, J. (2020). The ethnography of the global after globalization. *HAU: Journal of Ethnographic Theory, 10*(3), 1042–1045. https://doi.org/10.1086/712095

Rutschman, A. S. (2021a). The COVID-19 vaccine race: Intellectual property, collaboration (s), nationalism and misinformation. *Washington University Journal of Law and Policy*, *64*. https://openscholarship.wustl. edu/law_journal_law_policy/vol64/iss1/12

Rutschman, A. S. (2021b). Is there a cure for vaccine nationalism? *Current History*, *120*(822), 9–14. https:// doi.org/10.1525/curh.2021.120.822.9

Sands, P. (2020, March 11). Coronavirus response must be 'never again'. *Financial Times*. https://www.ft.com/ content/c8eae26c-6204-11ea-abcc-910c5b38d9ed?fbclid=IwAR1pFeK6H5M5Di2C7nHA1lw0WKXBLOki 3WGcGzPjK4LGzIoekkuQmbpKLO8

Schlanger, Z. (2020, December 23). The mink pandemic is no joke. *The Atlantic*. https://www.theatlantic.com/ health/archive/2020/12/minks-pandemic/617476/

Sharma, S., Kawa, N., & Gomber, A. (2021). WHO's allocation framework for COVAX: Is it fair? *Journal of Medical Ethics*. Advance online publication. https://doi.org/10.1136/medethics-2020-107152

Sibal, S. (2021, May 22). EU parliament extends support to India-South Africa COVID-19 vaccine patent waiver. https://www.dnaindia.com/world/report-eu-parliament-extends-support-to-india-south-africa-covid-19-vaccine-patent-waiver-2891451

Storeng, K. T. (2014). The GAVI alliance and the 'Gates approach' to health system strengthening. *Global Public Health*, *9*(8), 865–879. https://doi.org/10.1080/17441692.2014.940362

Sweileh, W. M. (2017). Global research trends of World Health Organization's top eight emerging pathogens. *Globalization and Health*, *13*(1), 1–19. https://doi.org/10.1186/s12992-017-0233-9

The Guardian. (2021, February 13). No end to Covid pandemic without equal access to vaccine, experts say. https://www.theguardian.com/world/2021/feb/13/no-end-to-covid-pandemic-without-equal-access-to-vaccine-experts-say

The WHO Regional Office for Europe (WHO/Europe). (2020, November 7). Mink-strain of COVID-19 virus in Denmark. https://www.euro.who.int/en/countries/denmark/news/news/2020/11/mink-strain-of-covid-19-virus-in-denmark

The World Bank. (2011). *World development report 2012: Gender equality and development: Main report (English)* (World development report). World Bank Group. http://documents.worldbank.org/curated/en/ 492221468136792185/Main-report

United Nations Children's Emergency Fund (UNICEF). (2021). COVAX: Ensuring global equitable access to COVID-19 vaccines. https://www.unicef.org/supply/covax-ensuring-global-equitable-access-covid-19-vaccines

Usher, A. D. (2020). South Africa and India push for COVID-19 patents ban. *The Lancet*, *396*(10265), 1790–1791. https://doi.org/10.1016/S0140-6736(20)32581-2

Usher, A. D. (2021). CEPI criticised for lack of transparency. *The Lancet*, *397*(10271), 265–266. https://doi. org/10.1016/S0140-6736(21)00143-4

van Schaik, L., Jørgensen, K. E., & van de Pas, R. (2020). Loyal at once? The EU's global health awakening in the Covid-19 pandemic. *Journal of European Integration*, *42*(8), 1145–1160. https://doi.org/10.1080/ 07036337.2020.1853118

Velasquez, G. (2020). *The World Health Organization reforms in the time of COVID-19* (South Centre, Research Paper, 121). http://hdl.handle.net/10419/232245

Vezzani, S. (2010). Preliminary remarks on the envisaged World Health Organization pandemic influenza preparedness framework for the sharing of viruses and access to vaccines and other benefits. *The Journal of World Intellectual Property*, *13*(6), 675–696. https://doi.org/10.1111/j.1747-1796.2010.00400.x

Wahl, P. (2017). Between Eurotopia and nationalism: A third way for the future of the EU. *Globalizations*, *14* (1), 157–163. https://doi.org/10.1080/14747731.2016.1228787

Wang, A. (2021, June 24). China belt and road 'not ideological' foreign minister tells conference. *South China Morning Post*. https://www.scmp.com/news/china/diplomacy/article/3138562/china-belt-and-road-not-ideological-foreign-minister-tells

Wang, Z. (2021). From crisis to nationalism?: The conditioned effects of the COVID-19 crisis on neo-nationalism in Europe. *Chinese Political Science Review*, *6*(1), 20–39. https://doi.org/10.1007/s41111-020-00169-8

Weaton, S. (2020, May 18). Chinese vaccine would be 'global public good,' Xi says. *POLITICO*. https://www. politico.com/news/2020/05/18/chinese-vaccine-would-be-global-public-good-xi-says-265039

Whitehead, A. L., & Perry, S. L. (2020). How culture wars delay herd immunity: Christian nationalism and anti-vaccine attitudes. *Socius: Sociological Research for a Dynamic World*, *6*, 1–12. https://doi.org/10. 1177/2378023120977727

Wong, W. K. O. (2021). Sino-Western rivalry in the COVID-19 'vaccine wars': A race to the bottom? *Asian Education and Development Studies*. Advance online publication. https://doi.org/10.1108/AEDS-12-2020-0271

World Health Organization (WHO). (2016). A R&D blueprint for action to prevent epidemics. https://www.who.int/blueprint/about/r_d_blueprint_plan_of_action.pdf

World Health Organization (WHO). (2020a, April 24). Commitment and call to action: Global collaboration to accelerate new COVID-19 health technologies. https://www.who.int/news/item/24-04-2020-commitment-and-call-to-action-global-collaboration-to-accelerate-new-covid-19-health-technologies

World Health Organization (WHO). (2020b, August 6). The COVAX facility: Global procurement for COVID-19 vaccines. https://www.who.int/docs/default-source/coronaviruse/act-accelerator/covax/covax-facility-background.pdf?sfvrsn=810d3c22_2

World Health Organization (WHO). (2021a, January 18). WHO Director-General's opening remarks at 148th session of the Executive Board. https://www.who.int/director-general/speeches/detail/who-director-general-s-opening-remarks-at-148th-session-of-the-executive-board

World Health Organization (WHO). (2021b, May 11). Access to COVID-19 tools funding commitment tracker. https://www.who.int/publications/m/item/access-to-covid-19-tools-tracker

Yang, X. (2021). US-China crossroads ahead: Perils and opportunities for Biden. *The Washington Quarterly*, *44*(1), 129–153. https://doi.org/10.1080/0163660X.2021.1894723

Zhong, R., & Schuetze, C. F. (2021, June 16). Taiwan wants German vaccines. China may be standing in its way. *New York Times*. https://www.nytimes.com/2021/06/16/business/taiwan-china-biontech-vaccine.html

Zhou, Y. R., & Coleman, W. D. (2016). Accelerated contagion and response: Understanding the relationships among globalization, time, and disease. *Globalizations*, *13*(3), 285–299. https://doi.org/10.1080/14747731.2015.1056498

India's pandemic: spectacle, social murder and authoritarian politics in a lockdown nation

Alf Gunvald Nilsen ⓘ

ABSTRACT
This article maps and analyses the trajectory of India's Covid-19 pandemic from its onset in early 2020 until the outbreak of the country's devastating second wave a little over a year later. I begin with a critique of the lockdown policy of the right-wing Hindu nationalist government of the Bharatiya Janata Party (BJP) and Prime Minister Narendra Modi, which served as a political spectacle rather than a public health intervention. I then proceed to detail how India as a lockdown nation witnessed forms of social suffering and political repression that can only be truly understood in light of how the trajectory and impact of the COVID-19 pandemic was shaped by two preexisting crises in India's economy and polity. In conclusion, I reflect on the likely political outcomes of the pandemic, considering both the impact of its second wave, and the emergence of oppositional sociopolitical forces in the country.

Introduction

On 31 December 2019, when China first alerted the World Health Organization (WHO) about several cases of unusual pneumonia in the port city of Wuhan, India was in the throes of one of the largest protest movements the country had witnessed since Narendra Modi and the right-wing Hindu nationalist Bharatiya Janata Party (BJP) first took power in 2014. Hundreds of thousands of people were out on the streets, from Punjab in the north to Tamil Nadu in the south, protesting against the Citizenship Amendment Act (CAA) that had been passed into law in the first week of December that year. As activists rightly pointed out, the CAA threatens to make Muslims second-class citizens in their own country, and at this point in time, the Indian nation – the world's largest democracy – looked set to face a 2020 that would be defined by a contest over the future of secular constitutionalism (see Nilsen, 2020a).

As we now know, things turned out very differently. India reported its first case of COVID-19 on 30 January 2020 – the patient was a student who had returned from Wuhan to the southern Indian state of Kerala. In the first week of February, three more cases were reported, and a month later, another 22 cases were confirmed. By the middle of the month, there were more than a hundred confirmed cases in the country (see Ray & Subramanian, 2020a). By that point in time, the WHO had declared that COVID-19 was a global pandemic, but the response from Indian authorities was, if anything timid: a COVID-19 awareness programme was launched in early March, but the Modi government persisted in claiming that community transmission was not a problem, and testing and tracing was only implemented to a very limited extent (Krishnan, 2020a, 2020b). In fact, on 13 March, India's Health Ministry issued an official statement that Covid-19 was not a health emergency, and that the Indian public had no reason to panic (The Hindu, 2020).

Then, on 24 March, Narendra Modi and his government did an about-turn and introduced one of the world's strictest national lockdown policies (see Nilsen, 2020b; Ray & Subramanian, 2020a, 2020b). A 1.3 billion-strong population was given all of four hours to prepare for an unprecedented disruption of everyday life, involving, among other things, a sudden and comprehensive cessation of economic activities. 'The nation will have to certainly pay an economic cost because of this lockdown. However, to save the life of each and every Indian is our top most priority', Modi said in his address to the nation. 'Hence, it is my plea to you to continue staying wherever you are right now in the country' (cited in Nilsen, 2020b). India, in other words, had become a lockdown nation. And over the next eight months, this lockdown nation would witness forms of social suffering and political repression that can only be truly understood in light of how the trajectory and impact of the COVID-19 pandemic was shaped by two preexisting crises in India's economy and polity (see Sundar & Nilsen, 2020).

These crises have different temporalities: one is a crisis of social reproduction and subsistence for the country's working poor, rooted in the long-term contradictions of India's neoliberal accumulation strategies; the other is a crisis of India's secular and constitutional democracy, which is brought about by the authoritarian populism of Narendra Modi's regime. In this essay, I offer an analysis of how the COVID-19 pandemic and the national lockdown intertwined with and amplified this dual crisis. I begin with a discussion of the fact that India's lockdown was not used to expand and bolster India's medical infrastructure. I argue that this has to be understood in terms of how the lockdown served as a form of spectacle, intended to project a public image of Modi as a strongman leader capable of swift action to defend Indian citizens against the pandemic, and argue that this has to be understood in terms of the political logic of Modi's authoritarian populism. I then move on to discuss the socioeconomic impact of the pandemic and the lockdown, with a particular focus on how the working poor were affected. I argue that the acute collapse of subsistence and social reproduction witnessed among the working poor lays bare how India's economy functions as a machinery for what Friedrich Engels (1844/2009) once described as social murder. In the third part of the essay, I survey political repression in the lockdown nation. More specifically, I show how the Modi regime has engaged in a war on dissent targeting, in particular, anti-CAA activists, and discuss how this relates to the political logic of the BJP's hegemonic project. In the conclusion, I reflect on prospects for post-Covid transformations in India in light of both the devastating second wave of the pandemic, which ripped through the country from March 2021 with almost unfathomable ferocity, and the emergence of the farmers' protest movement as a significant oppositional social force in the country.

Lockdown as spectacle

There is little doubt that the national lockdown that was imposed in late March 2020 failed to avert a public health crisis during the first wave of India's pandemic. In September 2020, India overtook Brazil in terms of the number of total cases, ranking second only to the USA (Firstpost, 2020). We do well to bear in mind, of course, that India has one of the lowest testing rates in the world, which means that the numbers that were reported at this time very likely to be underestimates (Naqvi & Kay, 2020; Saxena, 2020). In short, India became a pandemic epicentre. By early May, it was reported that India was doing far worse in responding to the pandemic and flattening the curve than its poorer South Asian neighbours. Compared to Pakistan, Bangladesh, and Sri Lanka, India had the highest cumulative and daily case count, and the highest death rate (Basu & Srivastava, 2020) (see Figure 1).

If we want to understand this dismal scenario, it is necessary to first consider the fact that the Modi regime – much like other authoritarian populist regimes – have responded to the pandemic with thoroughgoing disregard for medical expertise. 'The COVID-19 pandemic', leading health journalist Vidya Krishnan (2020a) observed on the eve of the imposition of the national lockdown, 'hits India as it is led by ideologues who have urged the use of cow dung and urine to prevent the spread of the virus'. The fact that motives other than acting according to the best medical advice available shaped the BJP government's response to the pandemic was quite evident from the early stages of the COVID-19 outbreak in India. Modi first spoke to the Indian nation about the pandemic on 19 March 2020, and used the occasion to announce a 'People's Curfew' – a one-day lockdown – on 22 March. Rather than addressing pressing questions related to public health and relief measures for those whose livelihoods would be most adversely affected by the pandemic, Modi exhorted citizens to do their patriotic duty by following government guidelines (Krishnan, 2020c).

Two days later, Modi declared a three-week national lockdown with only four hours' notice. The primary purpose of a lockdown is of course to flatten the curve of the pandemic – that is, to ensure a slower spread of the virus – in order to expand and strengthen the national medical infrastructure to cope with the increase in demand for treatment and care that will inevitably occur. At the time that the Indian lockdown was announced, health experts pointed out that the country had three weeks to prepare hospitals, convert stadiums into isolation centres, and procure as many ventilators as possible. The Modi government, however, did none of this (Krishnan, 2020a; see also Ray & Subramanian, 2020a). Indeed, as Jayati Ghosh (2020, p. 6) has pointed out, less than 0.04% of India's GDP was made available for immediate health expenditure, and less than half of these miniscule resources were distributed to state governments. It is worth bearing in mind that this failure took place in a country which ranks as number 184 out of 191 countries in terms of spending

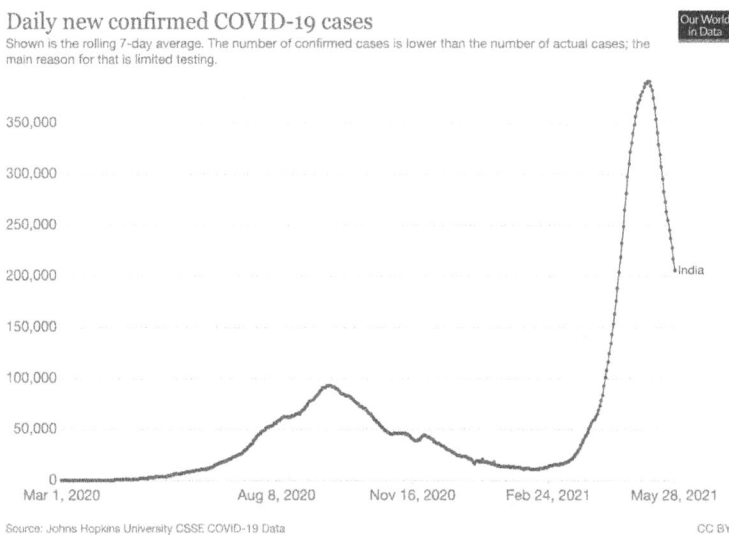

Daily new confirmed COVID-19 cases
Shown is the rolling 7-day average. The number of confirmed cases is lower than the number of actual cases; the main reason for that is limited testing.

Source: Johns Hopkins University CSSE COVID-19 Data   CC BY

Figure 1. The trajectory of India's pandemic, March 2020 to May 2021 (source: Our World in Data).

on public healthcare – in fact, India's annual public spending on healthcare is just above 1% of GDP, far less than its poorer South Asian neighbours. As a result of such systematic underspending, the country, according to the Brookings Foundation, had only 0.5 government hospital beds per 1000 people in 2017, which is highly inadequate even in the best of circumstances. There is only one public sector doctor for every 10,189 people, while the WHO recommends one doctor per 1000 people (see Nilsen, 2020b).

The lockdown was extended multiple times – from 15 April to 3 May, from 4 May to 17 May, and from 18 to 31 May – before a phased easing of restrictions began in June. It is revealing that the COVID-19 Task Force appointed by the Indian Council of Medical Research to advise the government was completely sidelined in the decisions to extend the lockdown (Krishnan, 2020d). In fact, just a few days after the third extension of the national lockdown, members of the COVID-19 task force openly stated to the media that the lockdown had been a failure because the government had failed to strengthen the country's medical infrastructure, and also had not expanded testing and tracing capacity (Krishnan & Konikkara, 2020; see also Krishnan, 2020e, 2020f).

So what purpose did the lockdown actually serve then? If we want to answer this question, we need to understand the centrality of spectacle in the political modus operandi of Narendra Modi and the BJP (see Nilsen, 2021c). The Modi regime, of course, is one of many avatars of the authoritarian populism that has become a political force across the North–South axis of the world-system during the past decade (see Hart, 2020; Heller, 2020). And, as is typical of authoritarian populism, the hegemonic project of the BJP hinges, to a considerable degree, on the figure of Narendra Modi as a strongman, linked directly to the people, opposed to both corrupt elites and threatening Others, and, crucially, capable of decisive action and leadership in the national interest. This image has been carefully crafted over a long period of time – arguably since Modi was chief minister of the western Indian state of Gujarat (2001–14) – and cultivated through multiple channels, including radio broadcasts, television, and social media (see Bobbio, 2013; Chakravarty & Roy, 2015; Rai, 2019). As Ravinder Kaur (2020a, p. 249) has argued, Modi's strongman 'brand' has been built, in no small part, through a series of 'attention-grabbing spectacles' that have become a core feature of the BJP's style of governance. Modi's 'signature quality', she proposes, 'is the capacity to make swift decisions – unilateral and almost entirely conducted in secrecy but released in the public domain as a thrill-inducing series of spectacles' (Kaur, 2020a, p. 249).

These spectacular policy decisions demonstrate to the public that Modi is indeed an undaunted man of action – someone who will intervene resolutely in the best interest of the people. The act of demonetization – the sudden withdrawal, in November 2016, of 86% of the cash circulating in India, supposedly to combat corruption – is one example of such spectacles and how they work. While demonetization did nothing to combat corruption and caused immense hardship to ordinary Indians, it nevertheless succeeded in building up Modi's image as a valiant warrior who would wield every weapon in the battle against corruption (see Ghosh et al., 2017). Similarly, the sudden imposition of a national lockdown was intended to project an image of Modi as a bold protector of the Indian nation in the face of the coming onslaught of COVID-19. These spectacles seem to defy the laws of political gravity – for example, as I show below, in another parallel to demonetization, Modi's lockdown policy did substantial damage to the country's working poor, who make up the majority of the electorate in India, but his approval ratings actually improved during the lockdown months (see Gettleman & Yasir, 2020; Kumar, 2020; Roy & Bellman, 2020). Ultimately, this reveals one of the most important strengths of Modi's authoritarian populism – namely that it is animated by what political scientist Neelanjan Sircar (2020) calls the politics of trust and belief. This is a form of personal politics, in which the people are asked to trust in the ability of a strong leader to make sound decisions for the nation. The politics of trust and belief contrasts, of course, with a more conventional politics of democratic accountability, in which citizens judge political leaders based on what they actually deliver. But it fits hand in glove with the designs of Modi's authoritarian populism, which peddles empty neoliberal promises of prosperity to India's citizens – some 60% of whom live on less than $3.10 a day – at the same time as it seeks to rally those citizens behind majoritarian designs for the making of a Hindu nation. In my concluding remarks, I ask whether this politics is still likely to be intact after the second wave of India's pandemic, which has revealed the inadequacies of Modi's policy response more starkly than ever. Now, however, I turn to an analysis of how and why the national lockdown did such damage to India's working poor.

A machinery for social murder

'Work just disappeared'. This is how 17-year-old plumber Vishal Kumar Maurya explained his decision to leave the metropolis of Mumbai for his native state Uttar Pradesh when the pandemic began to tighten its hold in late March 2020. Having spent most of his days since he arrived in the city six months earlier looking for casual work that would fetch him between 500 and 600 rupees as a daily wage, Vishal could no longer find anyone to hire him at the local labour junction. His only option was to return home: 'A virus we can fight but hunger we can't' (Daniyal et al., 2020).

Vishal was only one of many among India's 120 million migrant workers who did not abide by Narendra Modi's exhortation to stay put when the national lockdown set in. Instead, in a mass exodus of the working poor from India's cities, some 10 million people took to the national highways to walk home as their livelihoods disappeared without warning (see Ghosh, 2020; Singh, 2020). As I detail below, many embarked on their journey without sufficient food, and found themselves at the receiving end of harsh and humiliating treatment by state authorities. In Bareilly district in Uttar Pradesh, for example, a group of returning migrant workers were rounded up in a bus stand and hosed down with a disinfectant based on sodium hypochlorite, which is the main ingredient in bleach. Others were sent back to where they came from, as Modi's government ordered state borders to be sealed (Nilsen, 2020b). Some 972 migrant workers are reported to have died during their trek home, in road accidents and from causes such as exhaustion, malnutrition, and suicide (Mohanty, 2020).

The mass exodus was caused by the very structure of India's economy, where approximately 95% of India's workforce eke out a living in the informal sector, with low wages, poor working conditions, long working hours, limited access to social protection, and, crucially, insecure employment (see Agarwala, 2013; Barnes, 2014; Bhattacharya & Kesar, 2020; Breman, 1996; Ghosh, 2012; Shah et al., 2017; Shah & Lerche, 2020). When the Modi government imposed its draconian lockdown policy, economic activity ground to a halt, and informal sector jobs – particularly in manufacturing, construction, trade, and hotels and restaurants – were decimated (Anand & Thampi, 2020; Kapoor, 2020). According to media reports, unemployment in urban areas went up by more than 22 percentage points – that is, from 8.66% to 30.93% – between late March and the first week of April (Chishti, 2020; see also Menon, 2020). The result was 'severe economic distress' – and this distress was compounded 'by the fact that there was very little public assistance to prevent growing destitution and hunger' (Ghosh, 2020, p. 4).

There is no shortage of evidence of this destitution. For example, according to a survey of 11,159 migrant workers carried out three weeks into the lockdown, some 50% of those who had left the cities they worked in had rations left for less than a day; 96% had not received rations from the government and 70% had not received any cooked food; 70% of those walking home had less than 300 rupees left with them; 89% of those surveyed had not been paid by their employers at all during the lockdown (Stranded Workers Action Network, 2020). Two weeks into April, Indian media reported of growing hunger among migrant workers, who, due to the fact that they work outside their home states, were not able to access food grains from India's Public Distribution System (PDS).[1] This was despite the fact that, in March, the Food Corporation of India held 77 million tons of wheat and rice, which is three times the required buffer, and a bumper harvest was set to further swell public food stocks (Agarwal, 2020). A subsequent report from ActionAid India, published in August 2020, painted a similar picture of sustained distress: 81% of migrant workers and 71% of non-migrant workers in the informal sector reported losing their livelihoods; those who did not lose their work altogether frequently reported reduced working hours and less earnings, with many not receiving their cumulative wages in late March; many workers reported declining levels of food consumption, rapidly depleting savings, and, consequently, deepening indebtedness; many also reported having lost their housing as they were no longer able to pay rent (ActionAid, 2020). A recent comprehensive study from researchers at Azim Premji University further confirms this scenario: two-thirds of their respondents lost work, with casual and self-employed workers in the informal sector being hit hardest; those who did not lose their jobs outright reported huge losses in income – sometimes as much as 50%. Overall, earnings fell by between 40% and 50%, and 91% of poor households reported a loss of livelihood. As the report points out, this happened in a context where earnings were already very low, which means that the shock of the pandemic and the lockdown exacerbated food and consumption insecurity and deepened indebtedness. In fact, the vast majority of households surveyed reported reduced levels of food consumption during the lockdown (Kesar et al., 2020).

This reveals the extent to which India's economy is, most fundamentally, a machinery for what Friedrich Engels, in his study of the working poor in nineteenth-century England, called 'social murder' (Engels, 1844/2009). Engels coined the term to refer how the industrial working class confronted premature death as a result of how capitalist exploitation subjected workers to 'conditions in which they can neither retain health nor live long' (Engels, 1844/2009, p. 106). The workings of asymmetrical relations of power between capital and labour, he argued, 'undermines the vital force of these workers gradually, little by little, and so hurries them to the grave before their time' (Engels, 1844/2009, p. 106; see also Chernomas & Hudson, 2009; Grover, 2019). This becomes obvious if we consider in some detail the nature of what Stuart Corbridge and Alpa Shah (2013) have rightly referred to as the 'underbelly' of India's economic boom – a boom which began in the early 2000s on the basis of steadily rising growth rates since the early 1980s, and which averaged annual GDP growth rates between 7% and 9% throughout the 2000s, with only a minor and temporary dip after the financial crash of 2008 (see Chandrasekhar & Ghosh, 2015; Ghosh, 2012, 2015). What is striking about this growth trajectory, much of which has taken place after neoliberalization began in earnest in the early 1990s, is that it has failed to bring about a structural shift in the economy: India's economic growth, which has been driven primarily by finance, IT services and real estate, has failed to translate into employment growth, and labour's share of national income has fallen sharply (Chandrasekhar & Ghosh, 2015, pp. 5–11). And, closely associated with these trends, informal work continues to be the predominant source of employment in India (Bhattacharya & Kesar, 2020). As Chandrasekhar and Ghosh (2015, p. 18) point out, India's informal sector and its workers actually service the formal sector, and 'the low wages in the informal economy help sustain the formal sector profits' (see also Ghosh, 2015). Moreover, informal working relations are an integral part of India's growth process due to the fact that private employers in the formal sector are expanding their use of contract labourers with only the most minimal of legal rights (Chandrasekhar & Ghosh,

2015, pp. 18–21). In other words, India's informal economy is 'a major site of precarity' (Bhatta-charya & Kesar, 2020, p. 2) that has been reproduced and regenerated under neoliberalization, and which fails to adequately undergird subsistence and social reproduction for India's working poor (see Breman, 2016, 2019; Gooptu & Parry, 2015; Kannan, 2014) (Figure 2).

The workings of India's machinery for social murder becomes even more evident when we consider how the suffering of the working poor was aggravated by poor access to emergency relief and social protection under lockdown. ActionAid's (2020) survey of informal workers during the lockdown showed that 44% had not received any assistance with food, 75% received no cash assistance, and 85% of those who needed shelter did not receive it. In addition, many could neither access healthcare nor avail of state welfare schemes. This reflects, first of all, the fact that India has consistently failed to extend social rights to its poorest and most vulnerable citizens – a failure which has resulted in the country having far weaker social development indicators than those of poorer neighbouring countries such as Bangladesh, Pakistan, and Sri Lanka (Drèze & Sen, 2013). These consequences were worsened as a result of the 'extreme parsimony' (Ghosh, 2020, p. 7) of the relief measures that were announced during the pandemic and the lockdown (see also Nair, 2020). The first relief package that was introduced consisted mostly of budget items already committed to public spending prior to the outbreak of the pandemic and the imposition of the lockdown, and additional spending amounted only to 0.5% of GDP. An additional relief package was announced six weeks into the lockdown that supposedly amounted to 10% of GDP. However, close inspection reveals that the package mostly provided credit guarantees and other liquidity measures that did not necessitate fresh fiscal outlays. Total additional public spending therefore amounted to approximately 1% of GDP, much of which failed to reach those who needed it (Ghosh, 2020, p. 7). Above all, it was the 'inexplicable delay' (Ghosh, 2020, p. 7) in distributing food from the PDS that caused the most harm to the

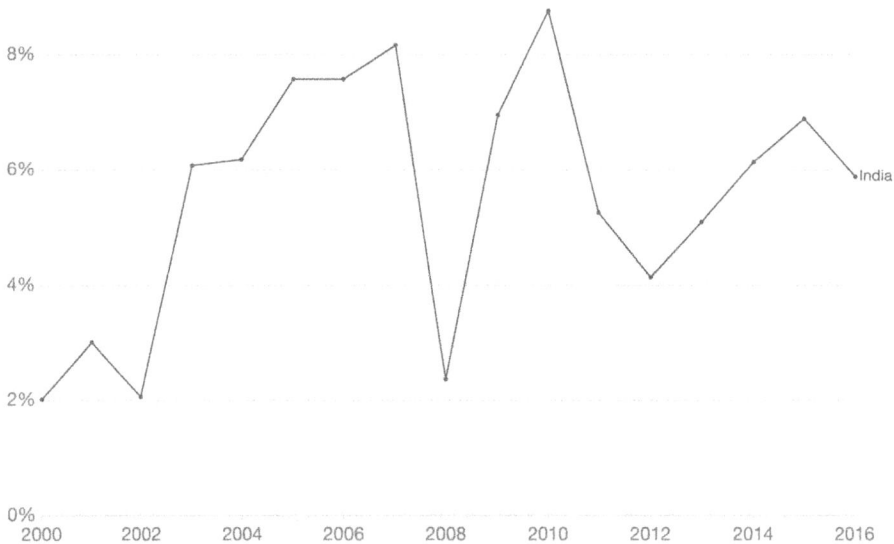

Figure 2. India's boom years: Annual aggregate GDP growth, 2000–2016 (Source: data.worldbank.org).

working poor (Indian Express, 2020; Varma, 2020). As with so many other facets of India's pandemic, the coexistence of plentiful food stocks and desperately hungry people was not a novelty: despite being a food surplus country, India ranks as number 94 out of 107 assessed countries on the 2020 Global Hunger Index, and is home to the greatest number of wasted children (low weight relative to height) out of all the countries assessed in the index (Upadhyay, 2020).

Interestingly, a similarly parsimonious approach characterized the Modi government's economic stimulus package, which in turn has long-term impacts on the Indian economy, far beyond the COVID-19 pandemic. Seemingly bound by strict neoliberal edicts, the government has been very reluctant 'to increase public spending beyond trivial amounts that are unlikely to do much to prevent capital declines in economic activity' (Ghosh, 2020, p. 8). A close reading of the stimulus package announced in the first half of May 2020, which the government claimed amounted to 20 lakh crore rupees, shows that direct fiscal stimulus would amount to less than 2.5 lakh crore rupees, or just a little over 1% of GDP (The Wire Analysis, 2020a). The majority of the measures were focused on credit and the easing of liquidity constraints for sectors of the economy badly affected by the national lockdown. However, in a context of declining demand, access to credit is likely to do little to improve investment, and banks and other firms are likely to use the available funds to balance their sheets (Ghosh, 2020, pp. 8–9). It is important to bear in mind that this failure to stimulate the economy through increased public spending happens against a longer-term backdrop of stagnation in the Indian economy. As Roshan Kishore (2020, p. 2) has shown in great detail, the Indian economy was 'caught in a prolonged deceleration even before the COVID-19 shock' (see also Nagaraj, 2020). In the quarter ending March 2019, the GDP growth rate stood at 2.5% less than the previous year, and by the end of March 2020, it had plummeted from 5.7% to 3.1% (Kishore, 2020). 'In a span of three years', Kishore writes, 'India went from being the fastest *growing* economy to the fastest *slowing* economy' (Kishore, 2020, p. 3). The COVID-19 pandemic and the national lockdown worsened an already dismal economic decline, as India witnessed a 23.9% contraction in economic activity from April to June 2020 (Singh, 2020). In July 2020, Oxford Economics, a global forecasting firm, confirmed the deficiencies of the government's policy as a further loss of economic momentum was expected in the third quarter. Overall, India has fared worst in all of Asia in terms of economic recovery, and is likely to take longest among major economies to regain pre-COVID-19 levels of economic activity (The Wire, 2020).

The Modi regime's unwillingness to invest in relief and stimulus contrasts sharply with its eagerness to push through further neoliberal reforms. In September 2020, the Indian parliament passed new legislation for the agricultural sector and introduced new labour laws. Both set of laws were passed in a great rush, and without much scope for discussion. In terms of agriculture, three new laws were passed – the Farmers' Produce Trade and Commerce (Promotion and Facilitation) Bill, 2020; The Farmers (Empowerment and Protection) Agreement of Price Assurance and Farm Services Bill, 2020; and The Essential Commodities (Amendment) Bill, 2020. Tweeting after the bills had been passed into law, Narendra Modi claimed that the new legislation will 'ensure a complete transformation of the agriculture sector as well as empower crores of farmers' and bolster his government's efforts to double the income of India's farmers. 'We are here to serve our farmers', Modi proclaimed. The new laws, however, work, first and foremost, to further liberalize Indian agriculture, and threaten to leave small and marginal farmers, who make up 85% of India's farming sector, at the mercy of overwhelmingly strong corporate forces (see Jawandhiya & Dandekar, 2020; Narayan, 2020; Nielsen et al., 2020; Sinha, 2020).

Aiming to put India among the top ten countries in the World Bank's Ease of Doing Business Index, the Modi government also rushed through substantial reforms of the country's labour laws:

44 central laws were subsumed into four broad codes of wages, industrial relations, occupational safety, health and working conditions, and social security. As critics have pointed out, these new labour codes will further expand India's informal sector workforce and leave many without the protection of formal contracts and benefits such as paid holidays and healthcare as labour laws will now apply to fewer firms, according to size and the number of workers they employ. For workers in India's formal sector, employment is likely to become more insecure while access to social protection remains very limited. Crucially, the new laws also severely curtail the capacity of trade unions for collective action (Sood, 2020; The Wire Staff, 2020b; The Working People's Charter, 2020).[2] Indeed, a crucial function the new laws is to signal to capital that the government is willing to confront labour (see Kaur, 2020b). Of course, as Varma et al. (2020) have shown, the laws fail entirely to address the needs of migrant workers, which became so evident during the national lockdown. Instead, the legislation deepens the informalization of Indian labour markets just as lockdown regulations are easing and desperate migrant workers have begun to return to the cities, willing, as Radhika Kapoor (2020, p. 6) puts it, to take up any work that comes their way 'even if the remuneration offered is lowered or the terms of employment are more precarious than before the shock of the pandemic' (see also Kumar, 2020).

In other words, instead of addressing the humanitarian crisis among the working poor, the Modi regime has instead pump-primed the machinery for social murder, and in doing so, the regime has also looked after the interests of Indian big business, which, as a class, has stood more or less uniformly behind Modi since 2014.[3] Indian capital, in turn, has done well during the crisis wrought by the pandemic and the lockdown. As Figure 3 below demonstrates, India was already a 'billionaire Raj' (Crabtree, 2018) before the pandemic. In 2019, the top 10% of the population earned 55% of all

Income and wealth inequality, India, 1951-2019

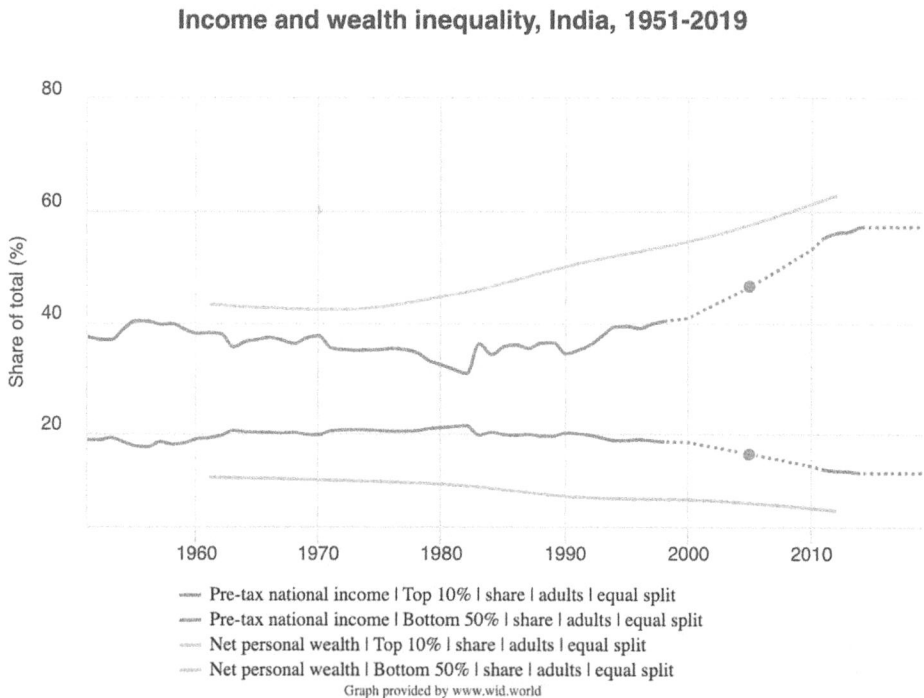

- Pre-tax national income l Top 10% l share l adults l equal split
- Pre-tax national income l Bottom 50% l share l adults l equal split
- Net personal wealth l Top 10% l share l adults l equal split
- Net personal wealth l Bottom 50% l share l adults l equal split
Graph provided by www.wid.world

Figure 3. Wealth and income inequality in India: 1951–2019 (source: World Inequality Database).

income and held 74.3% of all wealth (BQ Desk, 2019; Thakur, 2020; see also Chancel & Piketty, 2019; Himanshu, 2019). And between April and July, the combined net worth of Indian billionaires increased by more than a third – that is, their net worth increased by 35% to 423 billion US dollars (Kamdar, 2020; The Wire Staff, 2020c). India's capitalist class is also well-placed to further enrich itself as the Modi government, in addition to pushing through the new agricultural and labour laws, also liberalized investment regimes across multiple sectors of the economy, and dismantled environmental regulations that were widely viewed as impediments to industrial, mining and infrastructural projects (Haq, 2020; Zargar, 2020b).

In sum, then, what we have seen during the COVID-19 pandemic and the national lockdown in India is not only the amplification of the perverse workings of an economic structure that preys on the working poor through social murder but also a further consolidation of the power relations that produce these workings. As I show in the next section, these dynamics intersect, in the current perilous conjuncture, with a crisis in India's secular and constitutional democracy, which is brought about by the authoritarian populism that is at the core of the BJP's hegemonic project.

Authoritarian politics and the war on dissent

India is often hailed as an exceptional polity in the global South: since the coming of independence in 1947, the country's secular and constitutional democracy has remained remarkably stable and struck deep popular roots (see Jakobsen et al., 2019). This compares favourably, of course, to other regions and countries in the global South where democratic rule has tended to rest on feeble foundations and often has given way to outright authoritarianism (see Nilsen & Nielsen, 2016).[4] However, as India enters the third decade of the twenty-first century, Narendra Modi's BJP government has brought this democratic order to an unprecedented crossroads, and this has never been more evident than during the months that India has been a lockdown nation.

When the BJP came to power as the nation's governing party in the 2014 general election, it was, as already noted above, at the helm of a hegemonic project of authoritarian populism – that is, a form of conservative politics that constructs a contradiction between common people and elites, and then uses this contradiction to justify the imposition of repressive measures by the state (Hall, 1988). Initially, this project was constructed around a narrative of development that sought to address frustrated subaltern aspirations in the context of jobless growth while opposing dynastic elitism and promulgating individual entrepreneurialism. However, since the initial electoral victory in 2014, the politics of the BJP under Modi has increasingly come to gravitate around a majoritarian cultural nationalism that draws a line between true Indians and their enemies, and seeks to rally popular support for a crackdown on those enemies. Crucially, this line is defined in large part by religion – the ominous Other that authoritarian populism depends on in order to frame a unitary conception of the nation and national culture is, in Modi's India, the Muslim. Hate speech and vigilante violence against Muslims have escalated dramatically under the current government, and more recently, the precepts of Hindu nationalism have also come to be increasingly enshrined in law (see Jaffrelot, 2019; Jaffrelot & Verniers, 2020; Nilsen, 2021a, 2021b).[5] This hegemonic project has enjoyed considerable success – the 2019 elections saw Modi return to power with an even greater majority than in 2014, and 44% of all Hindu voters cast their ballots in support of Modi (see Nilsen, 2021a).[6]

However, it is not only India's vulnerable Muslim citizens who constitute the ominous Other in Narendra Modi's authoritarian populism. The enemy within also encompasses the political dissident who dares to question and challenge a government that claims to be acting in the interest of the people. This is evident in how the BJP government has waged a steadily escalating war on dissent in India. The first shots in this war were fired in early 2016, when student activists at Jawaharlal Nehru University (JNU) in Delhi were arrested on trumped-up charges of sedition (JNU Teachers' Association, 2017). The arrests helped spawn the idea that India confronts a threat in the form of 'anti-national' forces that are undermining the country from within. This idea has been used to justify a range of coercive attacks on dissenters – be they activists, public intellectuals, academics and students, lawyers, or journalists. Legal harassment and public vilification were the chief modus operandi of the state in the early stages of the war on dissent – for example, news channels that reported critically on the Modi regime have found themselves at the receiving end of police raids and investigations – but Hindu nationalist activists have also engaged in murderous violence against dissenting voices in the public sphere, as evidenced, for instance, by the assassination of journalist Gauri Lankesh in 2017 (Nilsen et al., 2019).

Modi's government began scaling up its war on dissent in late August 2018, when the homes of several human rights activists were raided in a nationwide police sweep. Five activists were arrested: Arun Ferreira, Sudha Bharadwaj, Varavara Rao, Gautam Navlakha, and Vernon Gonsalves. The arrests were linked to what is known as the Bhima Koregaon case. This case refers to the police investigation of violence that erupted in the western Indian state of Maharashtra in early January the same year. Dalit groups who had gathered to commemorate the bicentennial of the defeat of the upper caste ruler Peshwa Bajirao II by the armed forces of the British East India Company – a force that also counted a substantial number of Mahars (a Dalit community) in its ranks – were attacked by a Hindu nationalist mob. However, rather than scrutinizing the involvement of Hindu nationalist leaders in the attack, the police investigation targeted prominent activists who were arrested on charges of instigating the violence and planning a terrorist attack on Prime Minister Narendra Modi (see Nilsen, 2018; Shantha, 2020). And the crackdown did not stop there. Since 2018, altogether 16 arrests have been carried out in connection with the case – most recently, in April this year, of Dalit scholar and activist Anand Teltumbde, and, five months later, of Father Stan Swamy, a Jesuit priest who has dedicated his life to fighting for the rights of Adivasi (tribal/indigenous) groups in the state of Jharkhand in eastern India. The gravity of the charges has ensured that the accused have been refused bail and remain in police custody (see Jaffrelot, 2020; Mandhani, 2020; Nilsen, 2020c).

This strategy of imprisoning dissenters linked to draconian sections of the Indian Penal Code picked up momentum as the national lockdown began to quell India's public sphere. To fully understand the war on dissent in the lockdown nation, it is necessary to return to the scenario that this essay began with, namely the mass protests against anti-Muslim citizenship laws that shook India in late 2019 and early 2020. Often spearheaded by Muslims, this groundswell constituted the first substantial nationwide opposition to the policies of the Modi regime since it took power in 2014. Protesters faced brutal police actions and arrests, and Hindu nationalist mobs attacked student activists at JNU and groups of demonstrators elsewhere in Delhi. By late February this year, BJP leaders in Delhi incited mobs to attack Muslim neighbourhoods in northeastern parts of the city as part of their campaign against anti-CAA protesters. In the riots that ensued, 53 people – 39 of whom were Muslims – were killed, and hundreds of families were displaced from their homes. Despite the repression and violence, the protests continued until late March, when the national lockdown made it impossible to organize and mobilize on the country's streets and public spaces (see Nilsen, 2020c).

As protesters retreated, the Delhi Police, which reports directly to the central government and the Home Ministry under BJP supremo Amit Shah, swung into action, weaponizing the North East

Delhi Riots, and operating under cover of the national lockdown to persecute leading anti-CAA activists. At the heart of this persecution lies the claim, by the Delhi Police, that the violence in North-East Delhi was the result of a conspiracy carefully planned and executed by anti-CAA activists. The conspiracy, the police narrative goes, revolved around spreading misinformation about the CAA and the NRC, and then encouraging young Muslims to join in street protests. These subversive efforts allegedly reached their climax with the violent riots in late February, which the police claim were intended to cast India in a negative light in international media as erstwhile US president Donald Trump visited the country (The Polis Project, 2020).

The legal crackdown on anti-CAA activists began soon after the street protests had been cleared. For example, Meeran Haider, an activist and research scholar at Jamia Millia Islamia University and president of the youth wing of the political party Rashtriya Janata Dal, was arrested on 2 April on charges of instigating violent riots. Safoora Zargar, a media coordinator for the student activist committee at Jamia Millia Islamia University, was arrested a week later, also accused of instigating protests that escalated into violence in late March (Daniyal, 2020; Yamunan & Daniyal, 2020). Similarly, Devangana Kalita and Natasha Narwal, founding members of the feminist student collective Pinjra Tod, were arrested later the same month on charges related to their participation in the anti-CAA protests. After the two were granted bail, they were immediately rearrested on new charges that encompassed serious offences such as murder and attempted murder. Furthermore, the charges against the two were later expanded to include offences under the Unlawful Activities Prevention Act (UAPA) – a particularly draconian anti-terrorism law (Maniktala, 2020).

As the independent research organization The Polis Project (2020) points out in a detailed report, the strategy of the Delhi Police – which, according to Amnesty International, was complicit in the riots in North East Delhi – has been to begin by detaining and arresting junior activists from the anti-CAA protests young Muslim men from the communities affected by rioting. More than a month after the national lockdown had first been declared, residents of North East Delhi reported that police forces would sweep through their neighbourhoods to make arrests. 'If they could not find the person they were looking for', Divya Trivedi (2020a) writes, 'they picked up his family members and detained them until the person they were after appeared before them'. Their interrogations were then used to build evidence that was used to arrest and bring charges against more senior activists:

> During the interrogations, the young men are put under severe pressure to act as "witnesses" and produce statements corroborating the police narrative that the violence was caused by the anti-CAA/NRC protesters. In particular, the police coerce the youth to testify against senior activists in order to falsely implicate the latter in the violence. (The Polis Project, 2020, p. 22)

As the examples referred to above illustrate, the chargesheets that have accompanied the arrests of more senior activists tend to make very grave allegations without much substantial evidence. Indeed, there is much to suggest that what passes for evidence in these cases has been fabricated by the police to prop up the claim that anti-CAA activists were involved in a conspiracy to provoke violent riots. At the same time, evidence related to violence and incitement to violence by Hindu nationalists has either been suppressed or disregarded (Trivedi, 2020b).

The climax, so far, in this process – a witch-hunt by any standard – came in mid-September 2020, in the form of a 17,000-page chargesheet filed by the Delhi Police under the UAPA and various serious provisions of the Indian Penal Code against 15 prominent anti-CAA activists – among them Safoora Zargar and Meeran Haider, Natasha Narwal, and Devangana Kalita, all of whom had originally been arrested in April, and student leader Umar Khalid, who was one of the JNU students arrested on charges of sedition in 2016 (The Telegraph, 2020). The chargesheet, which also implicated renowned academics and leaders of national political parties as mentors of the arrested activists, was underpinned by two disclosure statements – effectively confessions – attributed to Devangana Kalita and Natasha Narwal. Interestingly, these statements were identical, despite supposedly having been made independently of each other, and on several pages, Kalita and Narwal had both clearly written 'I refuse to sign' in the margins (Mahaprashasta, 2020).

The purpose of these arrests is evident. It is, as The Polis Project (2020, p. 11) puts it, to produce 'a climate of fear that silences citizens by criminalizing dissent' (see also Nilsen, 2020c). And importantly, this war on dissent is joined at the hip with the majoritarian cultural politics of the Modi regime. During the COVID-19 pandemic, Indian Muslims have been scapegoated as super-spreaders of the coronavirus. This scapegoating seized on the conference of the Tablighi Jamaat – a Muslim revivalist organization – in Delhi in the second week of March 2020. Several attendees tested positive for COVID-19, and by the end of March, six conference attendees were reported to have died of the illness (Sebastian, 2020, Salam, 2020). At this point, Ziya Us Salam (2020) writes, 'the political establishment went into overdrive to paint the Tabligh, and by extension, the Muslim community, as responsible for the spread of COVID-19'. The political establishment was aided by a Modi-friendly media which wasted no time in peddling this narrative, and by the circulation of fake news on social media – a staple of Hindu nationalist politics in recent years (Trivedi, 2020c; see also Sinha, 2017). Such scapegoating aligns with the efforts of the Modi regime to produce a Hindu nation out of a secular constitutional democracy (Krishnan, 2020g). Most immediately, the stigmatization of Muslims as super-spreaders resulted in Islamophobic violence and harassment. There have been numerous media reports, for example, of Muslims being accused of engaging in 'Corona jihad' and being beaten up, while middle class neighbourhoods have implemented boycotts of Muslim street vendors (Ellis-Petersen & Rahman, 2020). As TIME journalist Billy Perrigo (2020a) puts it, it is quite obvious that all of this is 'exacerbating an already dangerous atmosphere for Muslims' in India.

Concluding remarks

If the trajectory and impact of the COVID-19 pandemic has provided us with a clear view of how India's economy is constructed as a machinery for social murder and how its polity is besieged by authoritarian political forces, it is only natural to ask where all of this leaves the Modi regime in relation to oppositional social forces. Does the BJP's hegemonic position in Indian politics remain intact after the pandemic has ripped through India, or are we likely to see a turning of the tide propelled by popular opposition to social suffering and political repression?

The initial lockdown months in 2020 witnessed some scattered protests by stranded migrant workers, and civil society groups played an important role in providing care and relief to those who made the trek from urban metropoles to rural homes. Trade unions opposed the new labour laws, and doctors and health workers objected to their working conditions (Sundar & Nilsen, 2020). Nevertheless, the politics of belief seemed to work its magic for the Modi regime: in late February 2021, the US firm Morning Consult reported that Modi's approval rating stood at 75% – higher than that of any other world leader tracked by the firm (Nilsen, 2021c). The question, of course, is whether the politics of belief will continue to ward off an hour of reckoning for Modi even as a second wave of the pandemic wreaks havoc on the country.

As I finalize this essay, India has been setting a new world record in terms of new Covid-19 cases every day for more than two weeks straight – that is, as of early May 2021, the 7-day average of new cases stood at 378,092, the cumulative case rate at 20,665,148, and the number of deaths at 226,188. These numbers doubtlessly underestimate the actual scale of the second wave of the pandemic. In fact, medical experts assume that the actual numbers of Covid-19 cases and deaths to be anything from five to thirty times higher than the official figures. This desperate situation reflected the fact, detailed above, that the Modi government failed entirely to address the Covid-19 pandemic as a public health imperative, despite the fact that it was warned by both parliamentary committees and its own medical experts that the country would be hit by a second surge in infections and that there were severe deficiencies in terms of supplies of oxygen and other medical necessities. In addition, the Modi regime's much trumpeted vaccination drive turned out to be a dismal failure due to inadequate manufacturing and procurement: only 2% of the population had been fully vaccinated at the time that this was written. Instead, Modi had declared to both national and international publics that India had succeeded in the battle against Covid-19 and directly enabled and pursued super-spreader events by giving the go-ahead to a massive Hindu festival and campaigning intensively for the state elections in West Bengal (see Nilsen, 2021d).

There is evident discontent and anger with the Modi regime as a result of this humanitarian crisis, and there have been numerous reports of dissent within the ranks of the BJP and the wider Hindu nationalist movement of which it is a part. However, this discontent will only be able to drive a progressive post-Covid transformation in India if it congeals with wider currents of protest in Indian society. This refers, above all, to the movement against the new farm laws that began to crystallize in October last year. Camped on the outskirts of Delhi since late 2020 in large numbers, the farmers' movement is widely considered to be a key node of opposition to both neoliberalism and Hindu nationalism (see Vanaik, 2021).

Now, protests by farmers are of course not new in India, and earlier generations of farmers' movements – especially the farmers' movements of the 1980s and 1990s – have been criticized for representing the interests of rich farmers, while marginalizing small and marginal farmers and agricultural workers (Banaji, 1994; Bentall & Corbridge, 1996; Dhanagare, 1994). In contrast, the current anti-farm law protests seem to be animated by a different configuration of social forces. As Shreya Sinha (2020) has shown in the context of Punjab, there has been active participation by farm workers' unions in these protests, and this is a result of activist efforts to build bridges between agricultural workers, most of whom are Dalits, and small and marginal farmers, who tend to be from dominant caste communities. Similarly, Sudhir Kumar Suthar (2018) has pointed out that the agrarian movements that are currently emerging in India are more diverse than what they used to be, and there is significant representation of small and marginal farmers, landless labourers, Adivasis, and notably, urban youth from rural backgrounds (see also Krishnamurthy & Aiyar, 2018).

This is not to say that caste and class differentiation are no longer issues in India's agrarian politics – as Sinha (2020) notes, the changing dynamics of organizing and mobilizing that she calls attention to have occurred within relatively clear limits. Moreover, a progressive political project would also have to extend solidarities to encompass the working poor in India's cities. The potential strength of doing so was amply demonstrated in late November 2020, when a nationwide strike brought together 250,000,000 workers and farmers in opposition to both the new farm laws and the new labour laws introduced by the Modi regime (Perrigo, 2020b). But again, building such solidarities would necessitate breaking with the binary political imaginary, central to much agrarian protest, that opposes an exploited rural India to an exploiting urban India (see Dhanagare, 2014). In sum, much hinges, therefore, on the ability of activists to extend and consolidate solidarities – not only between agricultural labourers, small and marginal farmers, and the urban working poor, but also between these groups, those subaltern citizens – especially Muslims and Dalits – who find themselves at the receiving end of an aggressive Hindu nationalism, and those voices who are in the line of fire in Modi's war on dissent. It was encouraging, in this regard, to see protesting farmers at the Delhi border demand the release of what they rightly refer to as political prisoners wrongfully charged under the UAPA. If there is to be a road ahead towards a progressive post-Covid future in India, it has to be built by fusing discontent with Modi's neoliberal Hindu nationalism with struggles against capitalist exploitation and with struggles for recognition, secularism, and democratic rights.

Notes

1. As both scholars and activists in India has noted, there were substantial problems with coverage in the PDS before the onset of the pandemic, with as many as 108 million people being excluded from its remit despite being eligible for subsidized grains (see Agarwal, 2020).
2. The new national labour laws were preceded by initiatives at state level to liberalize employment regulations (see Zargar, 2020a).
3. Indian capital shifted its allegiance to Modi and the BJP in a major way in the early 2010s, in part as a reaction to the Congress-led United Progressive Alliance passing legislation on land acquisition that was perceived to be a barrier to business, and in the context of declining growth rates and several high-profile corruption scandals. Corporate support has been crucial in funding the BJP's election campaigns in both 2014 and 2019 (see Nilsen, 2021a).
4. The only interruption in India's democratic trajectory was the Emergency period from 1975 to 1977, which was presided over by Congress Prime Minister Indira Gandhi (see Prakash, 2019).
5. This process of enshrining Hindu nationalism into law - a process which is best understood as Hindu nationalist statecraft - began with the abrogation of Kashmiri statehood in August 2019, continued with the Supreme Court verdict in the Babri Masjid three months later, and advanced further with the introduction of the CAA, the National Population Register and the National Register of Citizens in December the same year (Nilsen, 2020a). At state level, legislation against so-called 'love jihad' and cow slaughter is evidence of the same process (Nielsen & Nilsen, 2021).
6. The key factor that has enabled the BJP to win two consecutive general elections is the fact that the party has expanded its support base beyond its traditional urban middle class and upper caste constituency. Support for the BJP has increased strongly among the poor and among Dalits - India's formerly untouchable castes - and lower caste groups. This trend was already clearly evident in the 2014 general election, and was further reinforced in 2019, when the party increased its vote share from 34% to 44% among lower caste groups, from 24% to 34% among Dalits, and from 37% to 44% among Adivasis. Whereas the party increased its vote share across all classes, the largest increase happened among poor Indians – from 24% in 2014 to 36% in 2019 (Sardesai & Attri, 2019; Kumar & Gupta, 2019; Venkataramakrishnan, 2019).

Disclosure statement

No potential conflict of interest was reported by the author(s).

Funding

Research for this article was generously funded by the National Institute of the Humanities and Social Sciences and by the University of Pretoria Research Development Programme.

ORCID

Alf Gunvald Nilsen ⓘ http://orcid.org/0000-0003-4038-4400

References

ActionAid. (2020). *Workers in the time of COVID-19: Round 1 of the national study of informal workers.* https://www.actionaidindia.org/publications/workers-time-covid-19/

Agarwal, K. (2020). Coronavirus lockdown: As hunger grows, the fear of starvation is real. *The Wire.* https://thewire.in/rights/covid-19-100-million-hunger-pds-universal

Agarwala, R. (2013). *Informal labor, formal politics, and dignified discontent in India.* Cambridge University Press.

Anand, I., & Thampi, A. (2020). Locking out the working poor: India's inadequate response to Covid-19's economic crisis. *The India Forum.* https://www.theindiaforum.in/article/india-s-workers-lockdown

Banaji, J. (1994). The farmers' movements: A critique of conservative rural coalitions. *Journal of Peasant Studies, 21*(3–4), 228–245. https://doi.org/10.1080/03066159408438561

Barnes, T. (2014). *Informal labour in urban India: Three cities, three journeys.* Routledge.

Basu, D., & Srivastava, P. (2020). COVID-19 data in South Asia shows India is doing worse than its neighbours. *The Wire.* https://thewire.in/health/covid-19-data-in-south-asia-shows-india-is-doing-worse-than-its-neighbours

Bentall, J., & Corbridge, S. (1996). Urban–rural relations, demand politics and the 'new agrarianism' in Northwest India: The Bharatiya Kisan Union. *Transactions of the Institute of British Geographers, 21*(1), 27–48. https://doi.org/10.2307/622922

Bhattacharya, S., & Kesar, S. (2020). Precarity and development: Production and labor processes in the informal economy in India. *Review of Radical Political Economics, 52*(3), 387–408. https://doi.org/10.1177/0486613419884150

Bobbio, T. (2013). Never-ending Modi: Hindutva and Gujarati neoliberalism as prelude to all-India premiership? *Focaal, 67*(67), 123–134. https://doi.org/10.3167/fcl.2013.670109

BQ Desk. (2019). Rise in inequality in India second only to Russia, shows UN report. *Bloomberg Quint.* https://www.bloombergquint.com/business/income-inequality-in-india-rise-in-inequality-in-india-second-only-to-russia-shows-un-report

Breman, J. (1996). *Footloose labour: Working in India's informal economy.* Cambridge University Press.

Breman, J. (2016). *On pauperism in present and past.* Oxford University Press.

Breman, J. (2019). *Capitalism, inequality and labour in India.* Cambridge University Press.

Chakravarty, P., & Roy, S. (2015). Mr. Modi goes to Delhi: Mediated populism and the 2014 Indian elections. *Television and New Media, 16*(4), 311–322. https://doi.org/10.1177/1527476415573957

Chancel, L., & Piketty, T. (2019). Indian income inequality, 1922–2015: From British Raj to Billionaire Raj? *The Review of Income and Wealth, 65*(S1), S33–S62. https://doi.org/10.1111/roiw.12439

Chandrasekhar, C. P., & Ghosh, J. (2015). *Growth, employment patterns and inequality in Asia: A case study of India.* International Labour Organization. https://www.ilo.org/asia/publications/WCMS_334063/lang--en/index.htm

Chernomas, R., & Hudson, I. (2009). Social murder: The long-term effects of conservative economic policy. *International Journal of Health Services, 39*(1), 107–121. https://doi.org/10.2190/HS.39.1.e

Chishti, S. (2020). Urban joblessness up 22%, experts fear gains against poverty to be wiped out. *Indian Express.* https://indianexpress.com/article/india/joblessness-up-22-experts-fear-gains-against-poverty-coronavirus-6352143/

Corbridge, S., & Shah, A. (2013). Introduction: The underbelly of the Indian boom. *Economy and Society, 42*(3), 335–347. https://doi.org/10.1080/03085147.2013.790655

Crabtree, J. (2018). *The Billionaire Raj: A journey through India's new gilded age.* Tim Duggan Books.

Daniyal, S. (2020). Arbitrary arrests of CAA-NRC protesters point to political vendetta under the cover of Covid. *Scroll.* https://scroll.in/article/960619/arbitrary-arrests-of-caa-nrc-protesters-point-to-political-vendetta-under-the-cover-of-covid

Daniyal, S., Sharma, S., & Fernandes, N. (2020). As Covid-19 pandemic hits India's daily-wage earners hard, some leave city for their home towns. *Scroll.* https://scroll.in/article/956779/starvation-will-kill-us-before-corona-the-covid-19-pandemic-has-hit-indias-working-class-hard

Dhanagare, D. N. (1994). The class character and politics of the farmers' movement in Maharastra during the 1980s. *The Journal of Peasant Studies*, 21(3-4), 72–94. https://doi.org/10.1080/03066159408438555

Dhanagare, D. N. (2014). *Populism and power: Farmers' movement in western India, 1980–2014*. Routledge.

Drèze, J., & Sen, A. (2013). *An uncertain glory: India and its contradictions*. Princeton University Press.

Ellis-Petersen, H., & Rahman, S. A. (2020). Coronavirus conspiracy theories targeting Muslims spread in India. *The Guardian*. https://www.theguardian.com/world/2020/apr/13/coronavirus-conspiracy-theories-targeting-muslims-spread-in-india

Engels, F. (2009). *The condition of the working class in England*. Oxford University Press. (Original work published 1844)

Firstpost. (2020). COVID-19 in India and USA in infographics: A visual comparison of the situation in both countries. *Firstpost*. https://www.firstpost.com/health/covid-19-in-india-and-usa-in-infographics-a-visual-comparison-of-the-situation-in-both-countries-8802841.html

Gettleman, J., & Yasir, S. (2020). Modi's popularity soars as India weathers the pandemic. *The New York Times*. https://www.nytimes.com/2020/05/16/world/asia/coronavirus-modi-india.html

Ghosh, J. (2012). Accumulation strategies and human development in India. *Agrarian South: Journal of Political Economy*, 1(1), 43–64. https://doi.org/10.1177/2277976012001000104

Ghosh, J. (2015). Growth, industrialisation and inequality in India. *Journal of the Asia Pacific Economy*, 20(1), 42–56. https://doi.org/10.1080/13547860.2014.974316

Ghosh, J. (2020). A critique of the Indian government's response to the COVID-19 pandemic. *Journal of Industrial and Business Economics*, 47(3), 519–530. https://doi.org/10.1007/s40812-020-00170-x

Ghosh, J., Chandrashekhar, C. P., & Patnaik, P. (2017). *Demonetisation decoded: A critique of India's currency experiment*. Routledge.

Gooptu, N., & Parry, J. (2015). *Persistence of poverty in India*. Routledge.

Grover, C. (2019). Violent proletarianisation: Social murder, the reserve army of labour and social security 'austerity' in Britain. *Critical Social Policy*, 39(3), 335–355. https://doi.org/10.1177/0261018318816932

Hall, S. (1988). *The hard road to renewal: Thatcherism and the crisis of the left*. Verso.

Haq, Z. (2020). Govt unveils reforms to boost Covid-19-hit economy. *Hindustan Times*. https://www.hindustantimes.com/india-news/govt-unveils-reforms-to-boost-covid-hit-economy/story-BHGFUl8LanloIQ1rWoN5sK.html

Hart, G. (2020). Why did it take so long? Trump-Bannonism in a global conjunctural frame. *Geografiska Annaler: Series B - Human Geography*, 102(3), 239–266. https://doi.org/10.1080/04353684.2020.1780791

Heller, P. (2020). The age of reaction: Retrenchment populism in India and Brazil. *International Sociology*, 35/6(6), 590–609. https://doi.org/10.1177/0268580920949979

Himanshu. (2019). Inequality in India: A review of levels and trends. https://ideas.repec.org/p/unu/wpaper/wp-2019-42.html

The Hindu. (2020). Coronavirus | COVID-19 is not health emergency, no need to panic: Health ministry. *The Hindu*. https://www.thehindu.com/news/national/coronavirus-outbreak-union-health-ministry-press-conference-in-new-delhi/article31061163.ece

Indian Express. (2020). India lockdown: There's enough food, but India is struggling to get it to people. *Indian Express*. https://indianexpress.com/article/explained/heres-the-problem-theres-enough-food-but-india-is-struggling-to-get-it-to-people-in-covid-19-lockdown-6338645/

Jaffrelot, C. (2019). A de facto ethnic democracy? Obliterating and targeting the other, Hindu vigilantes, and the ethno-state. In A. P. Chatterji, T. B. Hansen, & C. Jaffrelot (Eds.), *Majoritarian state: How Hindu nationalism is changing India* (pp. 41–68). C. Hurst and Co Publishers.

Jaffrelot, C. (2020). Arrests in Bhima Koregaon case frame a transformation in India's polity and police force. *Indian Express*. https://indianexpress.com/article/opinion/columns/bhima-koregaon-case-stan-swamy-nia-chargesheet-naxals-6907744/

Jaffrelot, C., & Verniers, J. (2020). A new party system or a new political system? *Contemporary South Asia*, 28/2(2), 141–154. https://doi.org/10.1080/09584935.2020.1765990

Jakobsen, J., Nielsen, K. B., Nilsen, A. G., & Vaidya, A. (2019). Mapping the world's largest democracy (1947–2017). *Forum for Development Studies*, 46(1), 83–108. https://doi.org/10.1080/08039410.2018.1465461

Jawandhiya, V., & Dandekar, A. (2020). Three farm bills and India's rural economy. *The Wire*. https://thewire.in/agriculture/farm-bills-indias-rural-issues

JNU Teachers' Association. (2017). *What the nation really needs to know: The JNU nationalism lectures.* HarperCollins India.

Kamdar, B. (2020). India's rich prosper during the pandemic while its poor stand precariously at the edge. *The Diplomat.* https://thediplomat.com/2020/09/indias-rich-prosper-during-the-pandemic-while-its-poor-stand-precariously-at-the-edge/

Kannan, K. P. (2014). *Interrogating inclusive growth: Poverty and inequality in India.* Routledge.

Kapoor, R. (2020). The unequal effects of the Covid-19 crisis on the labour market. *The India Forum.* https://www.theindiaforum.in/article/unequal-effects-covid-19-crisis-labour-market

Kaur, R. (2020a). *Brand new nation: Capitalist dreams and nationalist designs in twenty-first-century India.* Stanford University Press.

Kaur, R. (2020b). Has Modi finally met his match in India's farmers? *The Guardian.* https://www.theguardian.com/commentisfree/2020/dec/10/modi-indias-farmers-government-factory-corporations

Kesar, S., Abraham, R., Lahoti, R., Nath, P., & Basole, A. (2020). *Pandemic, informality, and vulnerability: Impact of COVID-19 on livelihoods in India.* https://www.research-collection.ethz.ch/handle/20.500.11850/428008

Kishore, R. (2020). *Deceleration, pandemic, recession: Does India have a plan?* https://casi.sas.upenn.edu/content/deceleration-pandemic-recession-does-india-have-plan-roshan-kishore

Krishnamurthy, M., & Aiyar, Y. (2018, October 23). Reconceptualising farmer protests. *Business Standard.* https://www.business-standard.com/article/opinion/reconceptualising-farmer-protests-118102201234_1.html

Krishnan, K. (2020c). High on talk, low on substance: Modi's speech showed India is ill-prepared for COVID. *The Caravan.* https://caravanmagazine.in/health/high-on-talk-low-on-substance-modi-speech-showed-india-ill-prepared-covid

Krishnan, V. (2020a). Coronavirus threatens catastrophe in India. *Foreign Affairs.* https://www.foreignaffairs.com/articles/india/2020-03-25/coronavirus-threatens-catastrophe-india

Krishnan, V. (2020b). The callousness of India's COVID-19 response. *The Atlantic.* https://www.theatlantic.com/international/archive/2020/03/india-coronavirus-covid19-narendra-modi/608896/

Krishnan, V. (2020d). Modi administration did not consult ICMR-appointed COVID task force before key decisions. *The Caravan.* https://caravanmagazine.in/government/modi-administration-did-not-consult-icmr-appointed-covid-task-force-before-key-decisions

Krishnan, V. (2020e). Surge in COVID cases proves centre wrong; pandemic response marked by theatrics, not science. *The Caravan.* https://caravanmagazine.in/health/surge-in-covid-cases-proves-centre-wrong-pandemic-response-marked-by-theatrics-not-science

Krishnan, V. (2020f). Where pseudoscience is spreading. *The Atlantic.* https://www.theatlantic.com/international/archive/2020/08/amitabh-bachchan-india-coronavirus/615310/

Krishnan, V. (2020g). Modi government's targeting of minorities for COVID repeats old mistakes of HIV pandemic. *The Caravan.* https://caravanmagazine.in/health/modi-government-targeting-minorities-for-covid-repeats-old-mistakes-of-hiv-pandemic

Krishnan, V., & Konikkara, A. (2020). Members of PM's COVID-19 task force say lockdown failed due to unscientific implementation. *The Caravan.* https://caravanmagazine.in/health/members-pm-covid-19-task-force-say-lockdown-failed-due-to-unscientific-implementation

Kumar, S. (2020). Despite misadventures, BJP continues to enjoy widespread popularity. *Mint.* https://www.livemint.com/news/india/despite-misadventures-bjp-continues-to-enjoy-widespread-popularity-11600673794201.html

Kumar, S., & Gupta, P. (2019, June 3). Where did the BJP get its votes from in 2019? *LiveMint.* Retrieved October 10, 2019, from https://www.livemint.com/politics/news/where-did-the-bjp-get-its-votesfrom-in-2019-1559547933995.html

Kumar, V. (2020). Why India's migrant workers are returning to the cities they fled during the Covid-19 lockdown. *Scroll.* https://scroll.in/article/977275/why-indias-migrant-workers-are-returning-to-the-cities-they-fled-during-the-covid-19-lockdown

Mahaprashasta, A. A. (2020). Delhi police spreads riots 'conspiracy' net, drags in eminent academics and activists. *The Wire.* https://thewire.in/rights/delhi-police-riots-conspiracy-academics-activists

Mandhani, A. (2020). 2 years, 3 charge sheets & 16 arrests – why Bhima Koregaon accused are still in jail. *The Print.* https://theprint.in/india/2-years-3-charge-sheets-16-arrests-why-bhima-koregaon-accused-are-still-in-jail/533945/

Maniktala, P. (2020). What was the mysterious conspiracy of Delhi Police against Devangana Kalita? *The Leaflet*. https://www.theleaflet.in/what-was-the-mysterious-conspiracy-of-delhi-police-against-devangana -kalita/#

Menon, A. (2020). 90% workers lost Livelihood, 94% ineligible for govt relief: Study. *The Quint*. https://www.thequint.com/news/india/covid19-lockdown-economy-impact-construction-workers

Mohanty, B. K. (2020). Migrant deaths government won't see. *The Telegraph*. https://www.telegraphindia.com/india/coronavirus-lockdown-migrant-deaths-govt-wont-see/cid/1792114#

Nagaraj, R. (2020). Understanding India's economic slowdown: Need for concerted action. *The India Forum*. https://www.theindiaforum.in/article/understanding-india-s-economic-slowdown

Nair, R. (2020). Will centre's COVID-19 'relief package' really cost it Rs 1.7 lakh crore? *NewsClick*. https://www.newsclick.in/Coronavirus-COVID-19-Center-Modi-Govt-Relief-Package

Naqvi, M., & Kay, C. (2020). Questionable testing belies India's drop in Covid infections. *Bloomberg*. https://www.bloomberg.com/news/articles/2020-11-20/questionable-testing-belies-india-s-drop-in-covid-infections

Narayan, S. (2020). The three farm bills: Is this the market reform Indian agriculture needs? *The India Forum*. https://www.theindiaforum.in/article/three-farm-bills

Nielsen, K. B., & Nilsen, A. G. (2021). Hindu nationalist Statecraft and Modi's authoritarian populism. In S. Widmalm (Ed.), *Autocratization in South Asia*. Routledge.

Nielsen, K., Jakobsen, J., & Nilsen, A. G. (2020). Liberalizing Indian agriculture. *Terra Nullius*. https://www.sum.uio.no/forskning/blogg/terra-nullius/kenneth-bo-nielsen/liberalising-indian-agriculture.html

Nilsen, A. G. (2018). An authoritarian India is beginning to emerge. *The Wire*. https://thewire.in/politics/an-authoritarian-india-is-beginning-to-emerge

Nilsen, A. G. (2020a). India's breaking point. *The Polis Project*. https://thepolisproject.com/indias-breaking-point/#.X9NEnV5S_OQ

Nilsen, A. G. (2020b). COVID-19 and India's development crisis. *Paper*. www.nihss.ac.za/hssresponse

Nilsen, A. G. (2020c). Extreme Hindu nationalists smother dissent in India. *New Frame*. https://www.newframe.com/extreme-hindu-nationalists-smother-dissent-in-india/

Nilsen, A. G. (2021a). India's trajectories of change, 2004–2019. In V. Satgar & M. Williams (Eds.), *Democratic marxism 6 – destroying democracy: Neoliberal capitalism and the rise of authoritarian politics*. Wits University Press.

Nilsen, A. G. (2021b). From inclusive neoliberalism to authoritarian populism: Trajectories of change in the world's largest democracy. In M. Ray (Ed.), *State of democracy in India: Essays on life and politics in contemporary times*. Primus Books.

Nilsen, A. G. (2021c). Spectacle and social murder in pandemic India. *Boston Review*. https://bostonreview.net/global-justice/alf-gunvald-nilsen-spectacle-and-social-murder-pandemic-india

Nilsen, A. G. (2021d). India's Covid-19 disaster is a politically engineered tragedy. *Daily Maverick*. https://www.dailymaverick.co.za/article/2021-05-02-indias-covid-19-disaster-is-a-politically-engineered-tragedy/

Nilsen, A. G., & Nielsen, K. B. (2016). Social movements, state formation and democracy in India: An introduction. In K. B. Nielsen & A. G. Nilsen (Eds.), *Social movements and the state in India: Deepening democracy?* (pp. 1–24). Palgrave.

Nilsen, A. G., Nielsen, K. B., & Vaidya, A. (2019). Introduction – trajectories and crossroads: Indian democracy at 70. In A. G. Nilsen, K. B. Nielsen, & A. Vaidya (Eds.), *Indian democracy: Origins, trajectories, contestations* (pp. 1–12). Pluto Press.

Perrigo, B. (2020a). It was already dangerous to be Muslim in India. Then came the Coronavirus. *TIME Magazine*. https://time.com/5815264/coronavirus-india-islamophobia-coronajihad/

Perrigo, B. (2020b). India's farmers are leading one of the largest protests yet against Modi's government. Here's what they're fighting for. *TIME Magazine*. https://time.com/5918967/india-farmer-protests/

The Polis Project. (2020). Manufacturing evidence: How the Police is framing and arresting constitutional rights defenders in India. https://www.thepolisproject.com/manufacturing-evidence-how-the-police-framed-and-arrested-constitutional-right-defenders-in-india/#.X9SBll5S_OQ

Prakash, G. (2019). *Emergency chronicles: Indira Gandhi and democracy's turning point*. Princeton University Press.

Rai, S. (2019). "May the force be with you": Narendra Modi and the celebritization of Indian politics. *Communication, Culture and Critique, 12*(3), 323–339. https://doi.org/10.1093/ccc/tcz013

Ray, D., & Subramanian, S. (2020a). India's lockdown: An interim report. *National Bureau of Economic Research.* https://www.nber.org/papers/w27282

Ray, D., & Subramanian, S. (2020b). India's response to COVID-19 is a humanitarian disaster. *Boston Review.* https://bostonreview.net/global-justice/debraj-ray-s-subramanian-indias-response-covid-19-humanitarian-disaster

Roy, R., & Bellman, E. (2020). India vote shows how Narendra Modi is buffered from Covid-19 fallout. *Wall Street Journal.* https://www.wsj.com/articles/india-vote-shows-how-narendra-modi-is-buffered-from-covid-19-fallout-11605015673

Salam, Z. U. (2020). Hate in the time of a pandemic. *Frontline.* https://frontline.thehindu.com/cover-story/article31657319.ece

Sardesai, S., & Attri, V. (2019, May 30). Post-poll survey: The 2019 verdict is a manifestation of the deepening religious divide in India. *The Hindu.* Retrieved October 10, 2019, from https://www.thehindu.com/elections/lok-sabha-2019/the-verdict-is-a-manifestationof-the-deepening-religious-divide-in-india/article27297239.ece

Saxena, R. (2020). India's flimsy virus testing regime 'like flipping a coin'. *Bloomberg.* https//www.bloomberg.com/news/articles/2020-08-16/india-s-flimsy-virus-testing-regime-like-flipping-a-coin

Sebastian, S. (2020). After COVID-19 outbreak at Tablighi Jamaat conference, fake news targeting Muslims abounds. *The Caravan.* https://caravanmagazine.in/media/after-covid-19-outbreak-at-tablighi-jamaat-conference-fake-news-targetting-muslims-abounds

Shah, A., & Lerche, J. (2020). Migration and the invisible economies of care: Production, social reproduction and seasonal migrant labour in India. *Transactions of the Institute of British Geograpers, 45*(4), 719–734. https://doi.org/10.1111/tran.12401

Shah, A., Lerche, J., Axelby, R., Benbabaali, D., Donegan, B., Raj, J., & Thakur, V. (2017). *Ground down by growth: Tribe, caste, class and inequality in 21st century India.* Pluto Press.

Shantha, S. (2020). Case against Hindutva leaders ignored, no justice in sight for Bhima Koregaon violence victims. *The Wire.* https://thewire.in/caste/bhima-koregaon-violence-hindutva-leaders-case

Singh, K. (2020). COVID-19 has pushed the Indian economy into a Tailspin. But there's a way out. *The Wire.* https://thewire.in/economy/covid-19-india-economic-recovery

Sinha, S. (2017). Fragile hegemony: Modi, social media, and competitive electoral populism in India. *International Journal of Communication, 11,* 4158–4180.

Sinha, S. (2020). The Agrarian crisis in Punjab and the making of the anti-farm law protests. *The India Forum.* https://www.theindiaforum.in/article/agrarian-crisis-punjab-and-making-anti-farm-law-protests

Sircar, N. (2020). The politics of vishwas: Political mobilization in the 2019 national election. *Contemporary South Asia, 28*(2), 178–194. https://doi.org/10.1080/09584935.2020.1765988

Sood, A. (2020). The silent takeover of labour rights. *The India Forum.* https://www.theindiaforum.in/article/silent-takeover-labour-rights

Stranded Workers Action Network. (2020). 21 days and counting: COVID-19 lockdown, migrant workers, and the inadequacy of welfare measures in India. https://ruralindiaonline.org/library/resource/21-days-and-counting-covid-19-lockdown-migrant-workers-and-the-inadequacy-of-welfare-measures-in-india/

Sundar, A., & Nilsen, A. G. (2020). COVID-19 in Narendra Modi's India: Virulent politics and mass desperation. *The Wire.* https://thewire.in/health/covid-19-in-narendra-modis-india-virulent-politics-and-mass-desperation

Suthar, S. K. (2018). Contemporary farmers' protests and the 'new rural–agrarian' in India. *Economic & Political Weekly, 50*(26–27), 17–23.

The Telegraph (2020). Delhi riots: Police files charge sheet under UAPA against 15 for larger conspiracy. The Telegraph. https://www.telegraphindia.com/india/delhi-riots-police-files-charge-sheet-under-uapaagainst-15-for-larger-conspiracy/cid/1792180

Thakur, A. (2020). Top 1% hold almost half the wealth in India: Oxfam. *Fortune India.* https://www.fortuneindia.com/macro/top-1-hold-almost-half-the-wealth-in-india-oxfam/104013

Trivedi, D. (2020a). The virus of authoritarian strain. *Frontline.* https://frontline.thehindu.com/cover-story/article31542075.ece

Trivedi, D. (2020b). Crushing the right to dissent. *Frontline.* https://frontline.thehindu.com/cover-story/article31765280.ece

Trivedi, D. (2020c). Targeting a community. *Frontline.* https://frontline.thehindu.com/cover-story/article31374077.ece

Upadhyay, A. (2020). India is home to the world's most wasted children, as per the global hunger index 2020. *SwachIndia NDTV*. https://swachhindia.ndtv.com/india-is-home-to-the-worlds-most-wasted-children-as-per-the-global-hunger-index-2020-52022/

Vanaik, A. (2021). Farmers are leading India's biggest social movement in a generation. *Jacobin*. https://www.jacobinmag.com/2021/04/indian-farmers-strike-modi-bjp-social-movements-historical-struggles

Varma, D., Bharadkar, K., & Mehrotra, R. (2020). India's new labour codes fail migrant workers whose vulnerability was highlighted by lockdown crisis. *Scroll*. https://scroll.in/article/974137/indias-new-labour-codes-fail-migrant-workers-whose-vulnerability-was-highlighted-by-lockdown-crisis

Varma, S. (2020). Record harvest, record stocks; yet, why are people Hungry? *NewsClick* https://www.newsclick.in/Record-Harvest-Record-Stocks-People-Hungry

Venkataramakrishnan, R. (2019, May 1). 2019 results: BJP is no longer a 'Hindi heartland' party (except for Tamil Nadu and Andhra). *Scroll*. Retrieved October 10, 2019, from https://scroll.in/article/924468/2019-results-bjp-is-no-longer-a-hindi-heartland-partyexcept-for-tamil-nadu-and-andhra

The Wire. (2020). India economic revival worst in Asia, GDP growth to lose pace in Q3, says Oxford economics. *The Wire*. https://thewire.in/economy/india-economic-growth-gdp-covid-19-oxford-economics

The Wire Analysis. (2020a). Modi's Rs 20 lakh crore package will likely have fiscal cost of less than Rs 2.5 lakh crore. *The Wire*. https://thewire.in/economy/modi-rs-20-lakh-crore-package-actual-spend

The Wire Staff. (2020b). Explained: Here's why workers, opposition parties are protesting against the 3 new labour laws. *The Wire*. https://thewire.in/labour/labour-code-explainer-unions-strike-workers-opposition-parties

The Wire Staff. (2020c). Wealth of Indian billionaires rose by over a third during the COVID-19 lockdown. *The Wire*. https://thewire.in/business/indian-billionaires-wealth-rose-during-covid

The Working People's Charter. (2020). India's labour law reform: Briefing note for parliamentarians. https://workingpeoplescharter.in/media-statements/indias-labour-law-reform-briefing-note-for-parliamentarians/

Yamunan, S., & Daniyal, S. (2020). As Delhi Police crack down on student leaders, courts cite lockdown to justify lack of scrutiny. *Scroll*. https://scroll.in/article/960591/as-delhi-police-crack-down-on-student-leaders-court-cites-lockdown-to-justify-lack-of-scrutiny

Zargar, H. (2020a). Millions of Indian workers stripped of their rights. *New Frame*. https://www.newframe.com/millions-of-indian-workers-stripped-of-their-rights/

Zargar, H. (2020b). India's Modi dismantles environmental safeguards. *New Frame*. https://www.newframe.com/indias-modi-dismantles-environmental-safeguards/

Work in the post-COVID-19 pandemic: the case of South Korea

Kwang-Yeong Shin ⓘ

ABSTRACT
This paper addresses the transformation of work and employment in the period of post-COVID-19 in South Korea. The COVD-19 pandemic displays the failure of the market in managing the public health crisis and the crisis of neoliberal globalization, demanding massive state intervention to reproduce the stability of the social system. COVID-19 disrupted global production networks and global supply chains, generating economic disorder and mass unemployment. It also revealed the segmented labour market based on firm size, gender, employment status, and inadequate social protection. The COVID-19 pandemic, therefore, reveals problems that are embedded in the Korean economy, though at the same time provides an opportunity to discuss alternatives to the neoliberal economy. In particular, discourses on universal basic income and universal unemployment insurance have gained popularity as COVID-19 has disrupted mass' livelihood through promoting precarious work and expanding the population unprotected by labour laws and the social security system.

Introduction

COVID-19 has revealed doomsday scenarios of lockdowns, social distancing, and incessant mass hospitalization with mechanical ventilators. Furthermore, the coronavirus has disrupted the neoliberal economic order and, simultaneously, ordinary people's livelihood, thus engendering the foundation of the global capitalist system. It heralds the complete failure of the market in providing safety to the people and the return of the state in public health and the market economy.

COVID-19 brought about the shutdown of the national and global economy simultaneously from early 2020, shattering global value chains and the national market system. The coronavirus first erupted in Wuhan, China and rapidly engulfed the entire world within three months. From the beginning, there were disputes in many countries over the necessary policy responses to the virus. Unlike many countries in Europe that implemented lockdowns, however, the South Korean government did not impose lockdowns, and the impact of COVID-19 on the Korean economy was relatively less severe.

Nevertheless, the COVID-19 pandemic has typically disrupted the labour market in almost all countries, generating mass unemployment and shortening working hours in the manufacturing and service sectors. However, the prolonged COVID-19 pandemic has had differential impacts on workers and has amplified vulnerability in the labour market. Both disruptions of the global network of production and disturbance of local markets have destructive impacts on jobs and on work.

This paper addresses the changing nature of work and employment in the post-COVID-19 era in South Korea, exploring the breakdown of global production networks and the local employment system and the increasing precariousness of non-regular workers in the country. This paper argues that following the outbreak of the pandemic, further polarization and the marginalization in the labour market disclose the vulnerabilities of Korean society. The unemployment rate has decreased in spite of the mass unemployment as the unemployed have exited from the labour forces to become part of the non-working population. The latter displays the limits of traditional policy measures to mitigate the negative impacts of the pandemic on work and social security. As the platform economy emerges and the large size of the petty bourgeoisie persists, current labour market policies and social protections fall short in preventing social crisis. However, alternative policy discourses related to social protection, such as universal basic income (UBI) and universal unemployment insurance (UUI), have emerged from the economic crisis.

The COVID-19 pandemic and the economic crisis

The COVID-19 pandemic has resulted in a simultaneous reduction in both supply and demand. The outbreak of coronavirus in Wuhan and its spread to elsewhere in China in January 2020 led to a sudden disruption of China's global supply chains as Beijing halted factory operations across the country in the first week of February 2020. The lockdown of factories in Wuhan alone immediately affected the global auto industry as Wuhan is a supply centre of vehicle components for numerous global automakers (Williams, 2020). The breakdown of China-sourced global supply chains immediately led to a suspension of operations in Japanese automakers such as Toyota, Honda, and Nissan in China, and South Korean automakers such as Hyundai and Kia, GM, Renault-Samsung, and SsangYong in Korea (Hara, 2020).

Hyundai, the largest car manufacturer in South Korea, became the first global automaker to suspend production due to a shortage of hand-made wiring harnesses sourced from companies in China (Shin, 2020). Others such as Kia Motors, Renault Samsung Motors, and SsangYong Motor also suspended production for several days. This brought about mass unemployment in subcontracting companies and reduced working hours in South Korea.

Second, the disruption of companies' operations also occurred due to the Covid infection of workers in those companies in South Korea. Although the government did not impose a national lockdown, major automakers such as Hyundai, Kia, Renault-Samsung, and SsangYong repeatedly suspended operations for days at a time due to outbreaks amongst workers in those companies. In November 2020, the two largest electronics companies in Korea, Samsung and LG Electronics, also shut down their research labs and factories due to Covid outbreaks amongst their workers (Song, 2020; Yonhap, 2020).

Third, social distancing immediately affected the wholesale and retail industry, along with the accommodation, restaurant, tourism, and entertainment industries. People's everyday lives were immediately affected by the closure of schools, theatres, concert halls, gyms, religious organizations, and childcare facilities. Those who worked in those sectors lost their jobs or were forced to work much shorter hours than before. The service sector as a whole was thus heavily damaged by the Korea Disease Control and Prevention Agency's imposition of social distancing in 2020.

Strengthening segmentation of the labour market

In recent decades, there has been an ongoing transformation of the labour market in South Korea with regards to firm size, employment status, and work status. These changes have contributed to deepening of labour market segmentation along with the reshaping of wage distribution and working conditions.

First, there has been a segmentation of workers in accordance with company size. Known as the *chaebol*, large family-owned business groups in the manufacturing sector have grown into global corporations. They have globalized their production and sales via international markets since the late twentieth century. In contrast, small and medium-sized companies have maintained their conventional business practices. Labour unions were organized at the *chaebol* following the fierce workers' struggle that took place during the hot summer of 1987, with workers in the major industrial sectors demanding wage hikes and improved working conditions (Gray, 2008, pp. 52–70; Koo, 2001). As a result, sharp wage increases occurred in the key *chaebol* companies, widening the wage gap between large and small/medium companies. Moreover, as unions were concentrated in large companies, the union effect on wages has been substantial. Consequently, labour market segmentation by firm size became a significant new development in the post-1987 period.

The second moment of segmentation of the labour market occurred when the casualization of employment rose sharply after the financial crisis in 1997. Companies that survived the financial crisis pursued labour market flexibility by hiring diverse non-regular workers and thereby facilitating extensive workforce casualization. The proportion of non-regular workers increased by almost 10% between 2002 and 2004 (Shin, 2013, p. 343). The extensive casualization of work was an immediate outcome of an agreement among state, business, and labour to tackle the financial crisis in 1998 and its aftermath.

The third moment of the labour market segmentation was the employment system's polarization after the outbreak of coronavirus in 2020. The division of regular workers and non-regular workers has become wider as non-regular workers have seen massive layoffs. The proportion of those who were laid off after January 2020 was 36.8% for non-regular workers, compared to 4.2% for regular workers (Embrain Public Korea, 2021, p. 21). Furthermore, protected workers in the labour market have tended to enjoy stronger protections in public health than precarious workers. As the Korea Disease Control and Prevention Agency imposed social distancing to prevent the spread of the coronavirus, regular white colour workers in large companies and in the public sector were able to work from home. In contrast, non-regular workers were made redundant and laid off first due to the contraction of production and the market, except for indispensable workers necessary for essential services such as cleaning, care, and security. Ironically, those indispensable workers were the workers with the lowest wage and poorest protection in the labour market.

An immediate impact of the Covid-19 crisis was further fragmentation of the labour market by increasing the number of daily workers, i.e. the most precarious non-regular workers in South Korea. While the total number of non-regular workers decreased by 55,000, from 7.426 million to 7.371 million, daily workers on contracts of less than one month increased by 20.1% between August 2019 and August 2020 (Statistics Korea, 2020a, p. 23). Employers hired daily workers to enhance the flexibility of their employment system. Ironically, daily workers also show the highest unemployment rate among precarious workers, at 45.8% in 2020, compared to 40% for dispatched workers, 38.5% for atypical workers, and 38.3% for part-time workers (Embrain Public Korea, 2021, p. 51). Daily workers are the most precarious and are exposed to insecure work and minimal social protection. In 2020, almost 80% of daily workers were not covered by national pension and health insurance. Only 20.5% of them were covered by the national pension, 20.2% by health insurance, and 55.8% by unemployment insurance (see Table 1).

The petty bourgeoisie (jayeongubja), defined as the self-employed without employees, also increased as some unemployed workers subsequently became the petty bourgeoisie in the service sector. While the bourgeoisie who hire other workers (jabonga) saw a reduction of 2.1% between August 2019 and August 2020, the petty bourgeoisie increased by 2.5% during the same period. The petty bourgeoisie comprises a part of precarious social class since the majority of them are poor and are not covered by social protection. In 2020, the average disposable income of the petty bourgeoisie was 68.5% of that of regular workers, and the poverty rate, 16.26%, was almost three times higher than that of regular workers, 5.79% in 2020 (Statistics Korea, 2020e). The petty bourgeoisie also shows low social protection. More than half the petty bourgeoisie did not have any national pension coverage in place for their old age (Statistics Korea, 2020d, p. 34). Of course, they do not have unemployment insurance since they are self-employed. Thus, in 2020 the poverty rate of the petty bourgeoisie, 16.26%, is almost three times higher than regular workers, 5.79% (Statistics Korea, 2020e).

The recent labour market transformation has shown the rise of the NLFET: 'neither in the labour force nor in education or training'. While the NEET indicates those who are 'neither in employment nor in education and training', the NLEFT excludes the unemployed from the NEET (Serracant, 2014). The term 'NEET' was introduced to capture the non-working youth. However, the NLEFT may consist of diverse age groups, and thus is not necessarily restricted to young people aged 15–34. Some of those who lost their jobs temporarily exited from the labour force. Statistics Korea does not consider the NLEFT as part of the labour force and thus they are left out of the unemployment statistics. This leads to a paradoxical consequence. The economically active population decreased by 550,000 due to the economic depression after the WHO declared the COVID-19 pandemic on March 11, 2020. However, the unemployment rate decreased by 0.2 percent, from 4.4% in April 2019 to 4.2% in April 2020, and the employment rate dropped by 1.41 percent, from 66.51% to 65.1% during the same period (Statistics Korea, 2020b). An increase in the economically inactive population by 831,000 contributed to a lower unemployment rate. The unemployment rate declined further to 3.2% in August 2020 as most of the unemployed became part of the economically inactive population (Statistics Korea, 2020b). During the COVID-19 pandemic, a large part of the labour force has shifted from employment to non-employment, thereby leading to the simultaneous decrease in both the employment and unemployment rate.

Foreign workers

During the Covid crisis, many governments restricted labour mobility across national boundaries, thereby disrupting the global labour supply chains between developed and developing countries.

Table 1. Social protection by employment status in 2020.

	National pension (%)	Unemployment insurance (%)	Health insurance (%)	Union membership (%)
Regular workers	98.3	94.4	98.5	13.0
Non-regular workers	61.7	74.4	64.9	0.7
Dispatched	94.9	96.2	96.1	2.2
Daily	20.5	55.8	20.2	0.0
Part-time	77.6	81.1	79.0	0.4
Fixed term	86.6	86.2	93.1	1.2
Temporary	39.5	43.9	41.4	0.0
Home worker	80.2	76.2	78.7	2.5

Source: Statistics Korea (2020c, p. 29).

Thus, the pandemic damaged the weakest industries and workplaces that are heavily reliant on foreign workers. Since the outbreak of the pandemic, the supply of foreign workers to South Korea from China and Southeast Asia ground to a halt. While in 2020, 56,000 foreign workers were expected to come to South Korea, only 9.9% of them had arrived by August that year (The Ministry of Labor, 2020a).

Since foreign workers' wages are less than 30% of that of non-regular workers, the small and medium-size companies relying on low wages in the manufacturing, construction, services, agriculture, and fishery sectors have seen strong demand for migrant workers (Cho, 2010). The pandemic thus led to a sudden disruption of global labour supply chains, causing economic difficulties in those sectors. Employers have experienced serious labour shortages in the 'three-D jobs' characterized by dangerous, dirty, and difficult work. In response, on April 13, 2021, the Ministry of Labor announced the renewal of migrant worker visas for one year if they had exceeded their term of stay (Ministry of Labor, 2021a).

Foreign workers were exposed to the risk of infection because many of them live together at close quarters to save living costs and work in enclosed spaces. Some of them are illegal workers and thus are reluctant to visit public health centres even though they had Covid symptoms. Thus, some local governments issued an administrative order that all foreign workers should be tested for Covid at the public health centre in February 2021, provoking protests by civil society organizations as a violation of the human rights of foreign workers (People Power 21, 2021). Thus, the issue of foreign workers became an issue of the labour force, quarantine, and human rights.

Automation and precarious work

South Korea has the world's highest robot density in manufacturing. In 2018, it used 631 robots per 10,000 employees, eight times higher than the global average (IFR, 2018). This was an outcome of business' preemptive response to the growing labour movement in the 1990s. As the workers' movement grew in the summer of 1987, large companies took two strategies to respond to it. One was modular production development, by which large companies brought parts from small and medium-sized companies in South Korea or overseas via a vertical hierarchal network (Kim et al., 2011). The *chaebol* focused on assembling the final products, whereas small and medium-sized companies and offshore producers supplied the parts (Baek & Jo, 2009).

Another was the automation of assembly lines by introducing robots (Koo, 2000, pp. 235–236). During the COVID-19 pandemic, the 'un-tact' (a Korean term combined 'un' with 'contact') trend has accelerated robot automation in the service sectors, including office work. The banking sector and the education sector have also rushed to introduce un-tact services. Replacing face-to-face services, companies in the service sector could also utilize labour -saving machines such as vending machines In reality, employment in retail and wholesale, restaurants and accommodation, education, arts, and entertainment reduced by 10.2% between April 2017 and October 2020 (Song & Kim, 2021, p. 4).

The Covid-19 pandemic's impact was not so damaging to the manufacturing sector in South Korea due to the existing significant level of automation. Figure 1 displays the impact of the financial crisis in 1997, the subprime mortgage in 2008, and the current Covid-19 pandemic on the change of employment in manufacturing industry and retail and wholesale industry. Automation resulted in the pandemic having a less severe impact on manufacturing production compared to previous crises. However, retail and wholesale lost more than 123,000 employees between April 2019 and April 2020 (Statistics Korea, 2020a, p. 11).

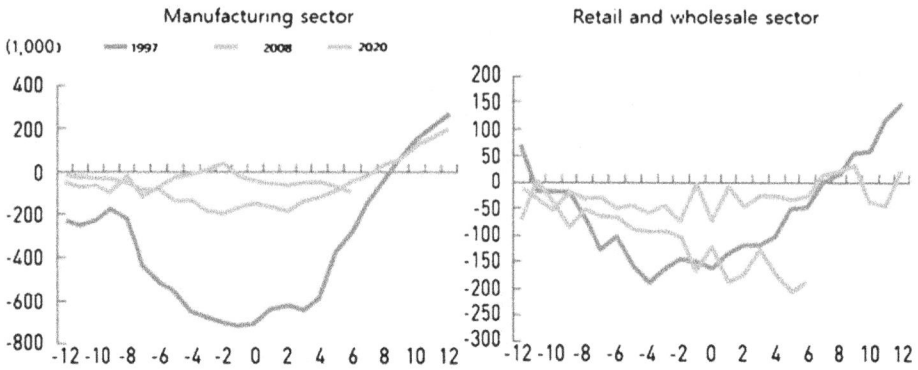

Figure 1. Changes in employment in the manufacturing industry and retails and wholesale industry for three crises. Source: Statistics Korea (2020). Press Briefs: Social Trends in Korea 2020, p. 16 (December 10, 2020). Note. The reference point is August 1998, May 2009, and April 2020.

As the Covid-19 pandemic persists, the application of robots and artificial intelligence in production and business will likely increase. An immediate result of the rapid transformation of industrial production and the service sector will thus be mass unemployment. Before the outbreak of Covid-19, the share of jobs at high risk of automation was estimated to be from 7% to 33% (Arntz et al., 2016, p. 33). The pandemic thus is likely to accelerate the application of automation and Artificial Intelligence (AI) as the un-tact economy becomes the new normal, thereby generating a significant change in the future of work.

Gender and work

The sharp decrease in employment in the service sector has affected female workers more than men as the former have been concentrated in the service sector. Here the service sector represents the contact (face-to-face) economy in which service providers meet customers directly. During the COVID-19 pandemic, the largest reduction in the number of workers occurred in the service sector. Compared with January 2020, the number of workers reduced by 367,000 in the food and accommodation sector, 218,000 in the retail and wholesale sector, and 103,000 in the private service sector in January 2021 (Statistics Korea, 2021). The impact of the COVID-19 pandemic has been thus much more severe for women in terms of layoffs and reduction in wages. The reduction in the women's employment rate was 1.5 times higher than that of men's (KWDI, 2020).

The closure of schools contributed to the reduction of women's employment since women had to care for their children at home (Kim, 2021). Thus, married women quit their jobs and moved into the non-economically active population. During the first wave of the pandemic, the probability of the transition from employment to unemployment for men increased from 0.65% to 0.75% between January and March in 2020, whereas it for women increased from 0.68% to 1.39% for the same period. The probability of the transition from employment to the non- labour force increased from 1.15% to 1.67% for men. In contrast, it increased from 3.09% to 5.09% for women (Kim, 2021, p. 65). The highest probability of the transition from employment to the non- labour forces was observed among the married women aged 39-44, mostly mothers of elementary school children (Kim, 2021, p. 67).

The shutdown of schools and the introduction of remote education via the internet could not attenuate the role of female workers as mothers significantly. The pandemic thereby revealed the severe unbalance between work and family life for women in South Korea, where mothers are still primarily responsible for taking care of their children. Care work for children has been focused on infants aged from 1 to 5. The pandemic thus shows that the current childcare system does not work well for elementary school children.

Alternative policy debates: rebuilding labour rights

The outbreak of Covid-19 reveals the lingering issues of labour rights again as the segmentation and polarization of work accelerates. The policy debate on basic income and universal employment insurance has emerged as the pandemic has disrupted the employment and livelihood of the people. Neo-liberal economic globalization has already undermined labour standards and labour rights achieved through past workers' struggles. In particular, the rise of platform workers has generated a new issue on labour rights. Platform workers are not workers in a legal sense, and are outside of the labour regulation and social protections associated with employment. They are not covered by unemployment insurance since they are not employed. They do not have a pension for old age either because there is no national pension scheme for independent workers. As a result, they must buy private insurance. In short, they are entirely uncovered by public social protections. The changes in the labour market generate incompatibility of existing social protection schemes with new forms of work.

As an alternative to social protection, the idea of universal basic income (hereafter UBI) has become popular in academic circles and in civil society in South Korea (D. Kim, 2020). The pandemic has contributed to the introduction of UBI as a means of overcoming the underdeveloped welfare state and the rise of the platform economy. Lee Jae-Myung, Governor of Gyeonggi province, advocated for UBI and started to discuss the UBI as the main agenda of his 2022 presidential campaign. He announced that the government gives 2,000,000 won ($1750) to the young people aged between 19 and 29 and 1,000,000 won ($875) to all other citizens every year.[1] Governor Lee already implemented the regional grant scheme on a smaller scale, granting payments to residents in Gyeonggi province alone.

The principle of the UBI as originally suggested by Philippe Van Parijs, was simple and was a way to promote real freedom for all to make their own choices. Freedom as a socialist ideal is a core value of his proposal so that the UBI should be unconditional, universal, and sufficient to meet basic needs (Parijs, 1995). In South Korea, discussions around UBI have emerged from the discourse on the welfare state as a policy response to poverty, rather than from socialist ideas. However, the COVID-19 pandemic has accelerated the debate. Governor Lee is also an influential politician, and the public have become familiar with the UBI scheme due to the experience of the disaster relief payments in 2020.[2]

Another approach to the deficiency of the social protection system has been to propose universal unemployment insurance (hereafter UUI), which covers the petty bourgeoisie and non-regular workers (Ministry of Labor, 2020b). Proponents of UUI argue that a large proportion of non-regular workers lies outside of social protection under the current system. In addition, the petty bourgeoisie, which amounts to almost 20% of the labour force, remain outside of the state's social protection if they meet with bankruptcy or poverty. They complained that they could not gain assistance from the government even though the pandemic significantly damaged their income.

Social policy debates have been intense during the elections ever since the transition to democracy began in 1987. Lee Jae-Myung is leading in the opinion polls recently, while other candidates from the ruling Democratic Party support the idea of UUI as an extension of existing social security programmes (Ki, 2020). However, proponents of insurance-based social protection have criticized UBI, arguing that it is not efficient in dealing with poverty and redistribution (Yang, 2020).

Oh Sehoon of the conservative People Power Party was elected in the local by-election of mayor in Seoul in April 2021, proposing an 'assured income' to transfer a different amount of money according to the level of household income.[3] Criticizing UBI as a populist idea, he proposed the assured income scheme, arguing that this would replace all public transfers to the poor. As such, this idea can be seen as a modified version of Milton Freedman's negative income tax (Choi, 2021).

Social policy responses to precarious work and life in the post-COVID 19 will be one of the most important issues in the next presidential election in March 2022. For the last three decades, the debates on economic policy have overwhelmed the policy debates in the presidential elections. The politicization of social protection is new to the Korean presidential elections, and thus, the next election will likely be a turning point in welfare politics in South Korea. This is significant, given the absence of a strong leftist party or influential labour unions.

Concluding remarks

The Covid-19 pandemic has posed a significant challenge to global capitalism. While it has been a health crisis, it has undermined the global economy and the lives of precarious social groups. South Korea, which had experienced other fatal pandemics such as the severe acute respiratory syndrome (SARS) and the Middle East respiratory syndrome (MERS) before, was effectively able to implement countermeasures.

Nevertheless, disruption of global production networks and the disorder of the domestic market led to the further polarization and casualization of work in South Korea. The suspension of production due to shortages of parts supply had knock-on effects on subcontracting firms generating unemployment and shorter working hours. The pandemic has reinforced segmentation between regular workers and non-regular workers. The shrinking consumer market has also reduced the size of the petty bourgeoisie in the service sector and has driven the unemployed into the inactive labour force.

The pandemic has driven female workers with children from the labour market and eventually from the labour forces. The closure of schools has forced married female workers to provide childcare, thereby lowering the unemployment rate directly. The transition of the unemployed to the non-working population resulted in a seemingly paradoxical reality: Though mass layoffs occurred, the unemployment rate went down. Mass layoffs in the service sector with female workers with children led to the rise of the NLEFT, those who are neither in the labour force nor in education and training.

The Covid-19 pandemic has also contributed to the rapid rise of platform labour in the service industry and has accelerated automation in the manufacturing industry. The application of labour-saving technology persistently undermines the labour market and social protection system. More than half of non-regular workers remain outside of such social protections. With the sharp rise of platform workers, platform work becomes a critical social and political issue in the post-Covid-19 pandemic.

As an alternative to the current social protections, the discourse on UBI has become prevalent in South Korea. While it was only confined to a small group of radical scholars before the pandemic, now politicians such as Governor Lee have adopted the UBI as a part of the political agenda. This proposal has become popular due to the experience of cash transfer as a disaster relief measure. Although the government's income support in South Korea is different from Parijs' philosophical premises, the UBI as a new policy idea is gaining more support than ever before. In addition, the 'assured income' as a conservative alternative to UBI was proposed by Mayor Oh who promised to carry out a pilot experiment in the second half of 2021. As such, the politicization of social policy represents a new stage of Korean politics.

Notes

1. Lee proposed the UBI with the new tax such as carbon tax and basic income tax (Yonhap, 2021).
2. For the last year, 109 academic papers were published in journals in social sciences and humanities in South Korea. Daily newspapers report scholarly debates on basic income and Governor Lee's comments on related issues.
3. Mayor Oh promised to carry out a pilot experiment with 200 households in 2021. The main idea of the assured income is that the state transfer half the gap between the median income and the household income to the low-income households. Therefore, the amount of transferred income differs according to the level of income among the low-income households.

Acknowledgements

I thank the anonymous reviewers for their comments on the earlier version of the paper. Especially, I want to express gratitude for Kevin Gray's editorial comments that were very helpful in the revision of the article.

Disclosure statement

No potential conflict of interest was reported by the author(s).

ORCID

Kwang-Yeong Shin ⓘ http://orcid.org/0000-0003-1678-2126

References

Arntz, M., Gregory, T., & Zierhan, U. (2016). *The risk of automation for jobs in OECD countries*. OECD Social, Employment, Migration Working Papers 189.

Baek, D.-J., & Jo, H.-J. (2009). Systemic rationalization and labor flexibility: Focused on the in-house subcontract of Hyundai Motor Company. *Journal of Industry and Labor, 15*(2), 349–383. (in Korean).

Cho, D. (2010). Wage differentials between foreign workers and domestic workers. *Labor Policy Studies, 10* (3), 56–86. (in Korean).

Choi, E. (2021, May 5). The designer of Oh Sehun's assured income "the poor get much, the rich get small … more money for those who work". *Joongang Daily*. (in Korean).

Embrain Public Korea. (2021). *The survey report on COVID-19 and the change in working life.*

Gray, K. (2008). *Korean works and neoliberal globalization.* Routledge.

Hara, Y. (2020, February 6). Honda and Toyota to keep Chinese plants closed over the virus fears. *Nikkei.*

International Federation of Robots. (2018). *Robots density by country.*

Ki, M. (2020, June 9). Presidential candidates from the ruling party divided into two parts, basic income and universal unemployment insurance. *Seoul Shinmun.*

Kim, D. (2020, June 13). South Korea mulls universal basic income post-COVID. *The Diplomat.*

Kim, J. (2021). Gender differentials in the impacts of the COVID-19 on employment and its implication. *Economic Prospect*, KDI (in Korean).

Kim, Y., Je, J. H., & Jeong, J. (2011). Modular production and Hyundai production system: The case of Hyundai MOBIS. *Economy and Society, 92*, 351–385. (in Korean).

Koo, H. (2000). The dilemma of empowered union in Korea: Korean Workers in the face of global capitalism. *Asian Survey, 40*(2), 227–250. https://doi.org/10.2307/3021131

Koo, H. (2001). *Korean workers: The culture and politics of class formation.* Cornell University Press.

Korea Women's Development Institute. (2020). *Women's employment crisis and policy issues in the post-COVID-19.* KWDI Brief 58 (in Korean).

Ministry of Labor. (2020a). A policy brief for an extension of stay of immigrant workers, April 13, 2020.

Ministry of Labor. (2020b). A roadmap of unemployment insurance for all, December 23, 2020.

Parijs, P. (1995). *Real freedom for all, what (if anything) can justify capitalism.* Clarendon Press.

People Power 21. (2021). Demand for stop of showing administrative activity by discriminating foreign workers, joint declaration for the day of abolition of racial discrimination. Retrieved May 21, 2021, from https://www.peoplepower21.org/Solidarity/1776371

Serracant, P. (2014). A brute indicator for a NEET case: Genesis and evolution of a problematic concept and results from an alternative indicator. *Social Indicators Research, 117*(2), 401–419. https://doi.org/10.1007/s11205-013-0352-5

Shin, J. H. (2020, February 4). Hyundai Motor halts production at local plants on parts supply disruption. *The Korea Herald.*

Shin, K. Y. (2013). Economic crisis, neoliberal reform, and the rise of precarious work in South Korea. *American Behavioral Scientist, 57*(3), 335–353. https://doi.org/10.1177/0002764212466241

Song, S. (2020, August 23). Tech industry on high alert as COVID-19 hits R&D, manufacturing facilities. *The Korea Herald.*

Song, S., & Kim, H. (2021). Scars in COVID-19: Three issues in the labor market. *Bank of Korea Issue Note 2021–18*, Bank of Korea.

Statistics Korea. (2020a). Press brief for the April 2020 employment trend, May 13, 2020.

Statistics Korea. (2020b). Press brief for the May 2020 employment trend, June 10, 2020.

Statistics Korea. (2020c). Press brief for the result of the additional labor forces survey by types of employment (August 2020), October 27, 2020.

Statistics Korea. (2020d). Press reports on the additional survey of self-employment and economically non-active population survey (August 2020), November 11, 2020.

Statistics Korea. (2020e). The panel survey of finance and welfare 2020 microdata.

Statistics Korea. (2021). Press brief for the January 2021 employment trend, February 10, 2021.

Williams, M. (2020, February 5). Coronavirus hits automotive supply chain in China and beyond. *Automotive Logistics.*

Yang, J. (2020). Why is basic income not a factor of the development of the welfare state? *Economy and Society, 128*, 58–77. (in Korean). https://doi.org/10.18207/criso.2020..128.58

Yonhap. (2020, November 18). Samsung, LG temporarily shut down research labs over virus cases. *The Korea Herald.*

Yonhap. (2021, July 22). 2,000,000 won ($1750) to the young people aged between 19 and 29. *Yonhap News Agency.*

A new deal after COVID-19

Thomas Pogge ⓘ and Krishen Mehta

ABSTRACT
The COVID-19 pandemic has revealed grave structural faults in our global institutional architecture. We argue that political energies should now be focused on three main areas where transformative reorganizations are realistically achievable. In global health, we propose that monopoly patents be complemented by health impact rewards as an optional alternative incentive for developing and supplying innovative pharmaceuticals. To slow global warming, we propose a common glide path for reducing *per-capita* emissions, with the option to compensate for temporary excess emissions by financing the achievement of additional emission reductions in poorer countries. For the global financial sector, we propose eliminating fossil-fuel subsidies, reintroducing Glass–Stegall, protecting the fair value of international natural-resource sales, and instituting an alternative minimum tax on corporations, financial transactions taxes and progressive taxes on internationally operating digital businesses.

We are living in the shadow of the COVID-19 pandemic – anxious about our families, our friends and ourselves, depressed by worldwide suffering and anxiety, upset by knowing that once more the poor and marginalized are worse affected.

As we are struggling to cope, we find ourselves wondering: could we have been better prepared? Can we become less vulnerable to predictable challenges such as COVID-19? This essay discusses three realistic and interrelated reform agendas that, if successfully pursued, would make our social world more stable and resilient. These agendas concern reorganizing the pharmaceutical sector, averting climate catastrophe, and promoting a global tax system that lessens corruption and inequality.

Other reform dimensions may seem more important: banishing the threat of war, for example, or enhancing democratic governance around the world. Our proposals are based on the convictions that, within the political space opened by COVID-19, they afford the best opportunities for real progress, and that their implementation would also advance peace and democratic governance. To use the present crisis as a spur for meaningful structural reform, we must spell out realistic steps for whose realization sufficient political support can be mobilized. More can be achieved than in ordinary times. We can squander this opportunity by failing to question existing practices and institutional structures. But we can squander it also by being too ambitious and hence ending up without any meaningful progressive reform, as arguably happened after the 2008–2009 financial crisis.

We are inspired by the New Deal reforms made possible by the Great Depression: Farm Credit Administration, Civil Conservation Corps, Tennessee Valley Authority, Public Works Administration, Federal Deposit Insurance, Securities and Exchange Commission, Federal Housing Administration, National Labor Relations Act, Social Security, Banking Act of 1935 and other important progressive reforms. In contrast to the 1930s, we now live in a much more globalized world where truly transformative change requires intergovernmental cooperation, perhaps organized through existing or newly created international agencies. To achieve such transformative change, we must conceive a schedule of plausible reform ideas and then mobilize concerted political support for it from farsighted politicians and from mature citizens energetically exercising their shared responsibility to promote moral progress for their own country and humanity at large.

We begin with the reform most directly related to the present crisis.

1. Reorganizing the pharmaceutical sector

COVID-19 draws attention to how conducive the rules and practices organizing health care are to a successful pandemic response. This question is especially pertinent to the pharmaceutical sector, which paradigmatically exemplifies the essential components of human progress: *innovation* and *diffusion*. We need innovations; and we need these innovations to spread and be used to good effect.

Pharmaceutical innovation has helped realize dramatic gains in health and longevity, with huge cost savings from reduced sick days and hospitalizations. We should evidently want it to be sustainable. But how should it best be funded, seeing that the cost of bringing new pharmaceuticals to market is extremely high relative to the marginal costs of supplying additional units?

Currently, commercial pharmaceutical research and development (R&D) efforts are encouraged and rewarded through the earnings innovators derive from sales of their branded products. These earnings largely depend on the 20-year product patents they are entitled to obtain in WTO member states under the 1995 TRIPS Agreement. Such patents give innovators a temporary monopoly, enabling them to sell their new products at prices far above manufacture and distribution costs without being underbid by rivals. Worldwide sales of such patented pharmaceuticals amount to about $550 billion annually or 0.6% of the gross world product. Another $250 billion are spent on branded generics, which can be sold at higher prices thanks to the name recognition they acquired during their patent period (IFPMA, 2017, pp. 51–53). Thus, pharmaceutical innovation is financed through high markups by early users of new drugs.

An obvious alternative is to cover the cost of innovation from public funds, on the ground that a healthy population and workforce are a common good. We propose doing this through a Health Impact Fund. Jointly supported by many countries, this Fund would invite innovators to register any of their new pharmaceuticals for participation in 10 consecutive annual payouts, each divided among registered products according to health gains achieved the preceding year. With these reward payments enabling innovators to recoup their R&D expenses and to make appropriate profits, the price of registered products would then be capped to covering merely their lowest feasible cost of manufacture and distribution. The innovator would also have to agree to its registered product going generic after its 10-year reward period, even if it still had unexpired patents. Some variant of quality-adjusted life years (QALYs), as widely employed and refined in recent decades, could be used as a common metric for comparing and aggregating health gains across diverse diseases, therapies, demographic groups, lifestyles and cultures. To reassure funders and/or innovators, a maximum and/or minimum reward per QALY could be agreed.

The Health Impact Fund is best conceived as a complement to the current regime, optional for innovators. It might get started with annual pools of $6 billion – less than 1% of what the world currently spends on branded pharmaceuticals, and obtainable if countries representing one-third of gross world product contributed 0.02% of their gross national incomes. This financial contribution would be offset by savings on registered pharmaceuticals and other health care costs as well as by gains in economic productivity and consequent tax revenues.

Innovators would remain free to fully exploit their patents in non-contributing affluent countries. This would give innovators more reason to register (lower opportunity cost) and affluent countries reason to join the funding coalition. Over time, the Health Impact Fund might grow – through economic growth in contributing countries, accession of additional countries, or agreement to raise the contribution percentage – and would then attract an increasing number of new pharmaceuticals.

A commercial innovator would develop and register a product only if it expected to make a profit over and above recouping its R&D expenses. There is some controversy over the size of such R&D outlays per marketing approval. The Health Impact Fund would throw light on this question by revealing at what level registrations settle. If, with annual pools of $6 billion, the Fund hosted about 20 products, with 2 entering and 2 exiting in a typical year, this would show that the prospect of $3 billion over 10 years is seen as satisfactory. For if innovators viewed this prospect as either windfall or hardship, product registrations would equilibrate to a higher or lower level. The reward rate on the Health Impact Fund is self-adjusting to track the true cost of achieving health gains with new pharmaceuticals.

There are three main reasons for adding the Health Impact Fund to the current regime. We can appreciate them by comparing the incentives it would provide to conventional patent incentives.

1.1. Allocation of innovation efforts

Pharmaceutical innovators motivated by the prospect of large markups tend to neglect the – mostly communicable – diseases specific to poor people. Thus, the 20 WHO-listed neglected tropical diseases together afflict over a billion people[1] but attract only 0.35% of pharmaceutical-industry R&D (IFPMA, 2017, pp. 15 and 21). Another 0.12% of this R&D spending goes to tuberculosis and malaria, which annually kill 1.9 million people.[2]

These devastating and heretofore neglected diseases are the ones against which the most cost-effective health gains can be achieved, and the Health Impact Fund would therefore motivate innovators to prioritize them. This would make it a valuable counterpart to the Global Fund, GAVI and MSF by making available to them, at very low prices, the novel pharmaceuticals they need. The Fund would also engender deeper and broader knowledge about such diseases and greater capacities for developing additional, more targeted responses quickly. Innovators would thus be much better prepared to supply or develop pharmaceuticals suitable for confronting emerging threats such as Ebola or COVID-19.

1.2. How pharmaceutical companies tackle diseases

The current regime motivates innovators to develop marketable products and then to pursue high sales at high markups. The Health Impact Fund would motivate them to develop effective products to be deployed strategically to reduce disease incidence as fast and cost-effectively as possible. Collaborating with national health systems, international agencies and NGOs, such an innovator would seek to build a strong public-health strategy around its product, involving diagnostics and other factors relevant to treatment outcomes, bolstered by real-time monitoring to recognize and address possible impediments to uptake or therapeutic success. Such an innovator's highest ambition would be to supply not many patients but few or none – after slashing the target disease. With little work left to do in the remainder of the reward period, it would still get credit for substantial health gains, triggering large payouts toward its next R&D project.

Patent rewards, by contrast, are tied to sales volume and thereby discourage the development of drugs, and also strategies for marketing drugs, which would lower the incidence of the target disease. Wall Street is quite alert to these disincentives and ensures that pharmaceutical companies are mindful of them also (Nocera, 2018). The Health Impact Fund is needed, then, to motivate innovators to fight communicable diseases – including COVID-19 – at the population level. The absence of such incentives heretofore helps explain why pharmaceutical companies have invested far more effort into developing new maintenance drugs, taken long-term for symptom relief, than into new vaccines, which generally offer the best prospects for disease eradication. With all our scientific sophistication, all the trillions spent on pharmaceuticals, humanity has managed to eradicate only one disease – smallpox – over 40 years ago.

1.3. Diffusion of innovations

Thanks to a large number of affluent or well-insured patients, the profit-maximizing price of a patented pharmaceutical tends to be quite high. A typical example is the hepatitis-C drug *sofosbuvir* (Gilead brandname: Sovaldi). It was introduced in the United States at a price of $84,000 per 12-week course of treatment while production cost was estimated at $68–136, roughly a thousand-fold – 100,000% – markup (Sachs, 2015). In poorer countries, *sofosbuvir* is much cheaper, but still unaffordable with the also much lower typical incomes there. Most people around the world cannot afford advanced pharmaceuticals – at least until their patents expire, which, with *sofosbuvir*, will start happening in 2028.[3] Millions suffer and die from lack of access to pharmaceuticals that could be mass-produced quite cheaply.

No such problem would arise with Health-Impact-Fund-registered pharmaceuticals, which would be available without markup from day 1. Yet, despite their low price, innovators would still have strong incentives to bring such products, in top condition, to remote and impoverished places, with clear local-language instructions and adherence support for patients and medical staff, because the Health Impact Fund enables innovators to earn more than the sales price from providing a product.

Doing so is morally required. It is also collectively advantageous, especially with communicable diseases, which would be central to the Health Impact Fund. By containing and ideally eradicating such a disease among the poor, we protect everyone from the threat it poses. By allowing pharmaceuticals against communicable diseases to be priced out of reach of the poor, we ensure that many avoidably remain sick and continue to spread the disease. We thereby often cause more dangerous drug-resistant strains to emerge, as patients – desperate and poor – take less than the full course of treatment or self-medicate with drugs in diluted dosage. Drug-resistant disease variants constitute a rising share of the disease burden and pose grave dangers to public health, including that of the affluent.

There is another way in which marketing under the current regime endangers even affluent or well-insured patients. When products sell at huge markups, then the incentive to promote sales is powerful. Pharmaceutical companies do this, energetically. Some such efforts are merely wasteful:

rival companies battle over market share with massive promotion campaigns that largely neutralize one another's effects. Or patients are given extremely expensive patented products that provide no benefit, or no more benefit than a cheap generic or natural remedy. But often patients end up taking inappropriate drugs: harmful to their health or less beneficial than some alternative product would be. These problems strengthen the third reason for creating the Health Impact Fund, which would condition rewards on actual health gains for patients.

1.4. The main inspiration behind the Health Impact Fund

The recent outbreaks of Ebola, swine flu and COVID-19 bring into sharp relief all three reasons for complementing the current regime: we have too little knowledge and know-how in regard to infectious diseases of poverty, we allow poor populations to be breeding grounds for new diseases and disease strains, and we lack incentives toward coordinated global efforts to contain and eliminate diseases. Such efforts must include the poor: we need good new treatments for the diseases of poverty and must ensure that all people have access to important pharmaceuticals and can use them to optimal effect.

The COVID-19 pandemic has intensified the long-standing complaint that pharmaceutical companies are putting profits over people. This complaint also indicts ourselves. We should not design the pharmaceutical sector so that firms are torn between profits and people. Profits should be aligned with human health, so that firms are doing well by doing good. If the purpose of the pharmaceutical sector is the cost-effective avoidance of morbidity and mortality, then that is what we should reward and incentivize. This compelling thought grounds the Health Impact Fund approach: rather than reward innovations in a way that impedes their diffusion, we should align rewards with each innovation's true value, of which diffusion is an essential part.

1.5. The Health Impact Fund's transformative power

While monopoly rewards turn innovators into jealous spies, scouring the Earth to find patent infringers who may be using their innovation without license, the Health Impact Fund does the opposite: it encourages innovators actively to promote *widespread* and *effective* deployment of their innovation for enlarged impact. Wider deployment can be promoted by adding one's innovation to a patent pool or by subsidizing its use among the poorest even below variable cost and more effective deployment by various means that help users get the most out of their product. Greater effectiveness, insofar as potential buyers care about it, also promotes wider use.

In this regard, the Health Impact Fund improves upon compulsory licensing which, relying on competing generic manufacturers to drive down prices, remains caught in the tension between price and promotion: the cheaper the product, the less incentive there is to bring it, in top condition and with appropriate care, to remote and impoverished communities. The Health Impact Fund avoids this tension by giving innovators a financial interest in both: affordability and widespread optimal use of their product. By assigning more value to the health and survival of poor people than what they can afford to pay, it truly ensures that no one is left behind.

The Health Impact Fund is superior to compulsory licensing also by not jeopardizing innovators' recovery of their massive R&D outlays. It is not smart to put commercial innovators on notice that, if any of their innovations is really important, then states may appropriate it with token compensation. Promoting access in a way that undermines innovation is no better than what we do now: promote innovation in a way that undermines access. Neither regime delivers what we want: abundant innovation *and* universal access. If we delink the price of pharmaceuticals from the fixed cost of R&D – as we should! – then we should also delink innovator earnings from the sales price. Innovation flourishes only if innovators can recover their investments and make a decent profit.

Reducing disease with pharmaceuticals is complicated and involves many stages – from research lab to patient care. All these stages and components are interdependent, posing a highly complex global logistics problem. Optimal progress requires not merely the solution of many disparate tasks but also harmony among solutions. Early decisions about conceiving and pursuing R&D projects should already anticipate the challenges of successful deployment: how to identify the patients who can benefit the most and, for infectious diseases, those whose timely treatment would do most to slow contagion? How to make the product reach and benefit patients in remote and impoverished locations? How to build a strong collaborative public-health strategy around the product? How to fashion the best plan toward eradicating the disease worldwide?

These great potential synergies suggest that the Health Impact Fund would give rise to actors who can optimally run an entire worldwide operation, R&D plus marketing. Some pharmaceutical firms are well-positioned to reconfigure themselves for this role. Other organizations may also be: certain NGOs and product-development partnerships. Open to all, the Health Impact Fund would, over time, bring forth innovators that really excel at achieving cost-effective health gains through a well-coordinated global strategy of disease containment.

2. Averting climate catastrophe

The looming climate disaster has obvious similarities with the COVID-19 crisis. Both dangers have a tendency to grow exponentially. Both threaten a global catastrophe from which individual countries or regions cannot safely insulate themselves. In both cases, plausible countermeasures require concerted international collaboration; individual countries and national governments have self-interested reasons to defect from the collectively optimal collaborative plan; powerful economic interests block the path toward a global solution; and innovation is a key element in any plausible and realistic solution.

This last parallel provokes the question whether it is foolish to use patent monopolies to reward green innovations, thereby inhibiting their use. When green innovations are expensive to use, rational producers of electricity, cement or steel may well decide to do without, since this decision's fallout is mostly externalized as the additional pollution harms other (including future) people and the rest of our planet.

It would be much smarter to reward green innovations on the Health Impact Fund model, through an Ecological or Green Impact Fund (Pogge, 2010). This approach makes sense when two conditions are fulfilled: use of the incentivized innovation serves a morally or socially desirable purpose, which makes public expenditure appropriate; and contributions to this purpose can be quantified for proportional disbursement. The Health Impact Fund fulfils the second condition through a general measure of health impact. An Ecological Impact Fund can fulfil it by employing a suitable metric of pollution averted, which assigns weights to the various greenhouse gases, pesticides, aerosol particles, plastics, particulate matter ($PM_{2.5}$) etc. Green innovators would be asked to allow cost-free use of their innovation in exchange for 10 annual reward payments proportioned to their innovation's ecological impact. A well-financed Ecological Impact Fund would promote widespread use of green innovations while also encouraging green R&D and guiding innovators toward the specific R&D projects that can yield the most cost-effective ecological-harm reductions.

Fast-spreading and highly effective green innovations can make a crucial contribution to sustainability. But in view of the monumental emissions reductions we must achieve rather quickly, and of the immense resistance mobilized by interested industries and fossil-fuel owners, we cannot hope that green innovations alone, conjoined only with economic rationality, will save us.

2.1. Diverging interests

Further reflection on how to avert the looming catastrophe should start from the question why so little was achieved in 40 years, even while the basic facts and dangers were well understood. A sound answer must acknowledge – contrary to much trite rhetoric about everyone sitting the in same boat – the great divergences in our needs and interests.

At one end, there are superrich individuals with substantial fossil-fuel investments, with yachts and private planes, air-conditioned accommodations and a wad of golden passports. They would incur serious costs if their fossil-fuel holdings became worthless and their carbon-intensive lifestyles were curtailed. And they would suffer little inconvenience from even a severe climate deterioration: they can continue to breathe clean cool air within their mansions, limousines, yachts and planes, can enjoy indoor ski resorts (there is one in Dubai's desert), and, if they miss the real outdoors, they can settle in Canada, New Zealand, Norway or whatever place offers the best conditions remaining. Such people, even if they care a few decades beyond their own lifespan, have little to worry about.

At the other end, there are poor people in lower-income, mostly tropical countries, especially those who cannot avoid the outdoors: peasants, construction workers, rickshaw drivers, delivery people, animal herders, fisher folk. They can do little to mitigate the threats they face: unbearable heat, ever more frequent and severe extreme weather events, spread of tropical diseases, coastal erosion, salinization of drinking water, increasing scarcity of food and water. Many are suffering gravely and dying prematurely even today; and things will get much worse in the decades ahead.

Economic rationality provides a classical solution to collective action problems involving differentially affected parties: those with more to lose should contribute more to averting the harm. Even subsidizing the less vulnerable, they would still realize a net gain.

This classical solution does not work for the climate problem. First, the market value of known fossil-fuel reserves is in the tens of trillions.[4] It would be difficult to raise such amounts to pay off existing owners.[5] Second, those most threatened by the impending climate catastrophe are mostly poor or yet unborn: even with their very survival at stake, they cannot mobilize large sums. Third, it would be morally absurd beyond words to ask present and future subsistence farmers in the tropics, who have barely contributed to the problem, to pay compensation to the world's affluent, whose actions have caused the climate emergency. Doing so would be akin to criminal extortion: 'unless you pay us, we will continue destroying the preconditions of your survival'.

2.2. A moral solution

Humanity's best hope for solving the climate emergency is a moral solution that limits future greenhouse gas emissions enough to avert catastrophe, allocates these limitations fairly among generations, and then allocates each generation's burden fairly among contemporaries.

Before addressing these conditions, let us add a fourth. There is also strong reason to prefer a solution that encourages relevant agents to focus their contributions on the larger, more cost-effective emissions reductions. The 2015 Paris Agreement fails in this regard by strongly focusing the attention of national governments on emissions emanating within their own borders. In the case of industrialized countries – the United States, Japan, China, Russia, and the European Union – this focus misses a lot. These countries should reduce their domestic emissions, yes. But it also matters greatly what construction projects their corporations are undertaking abroad, what such projects their governments and banks are financing or subsidizing, what principles and priorities are guiding their development cooperation and participation in international organizations (World Bank, IMF, G20, WTO, OECD, etc.).

To illustrate. Though still burning more coal than the rest of the world combined,[6] China is beginning to move away from fossil fuels in the spirit of the Paris Agreement. But, to utilize existing skills and capacities, and to preserve jobs, Chinese firms, banks and (national and provincial) governments are also collaborating to offer developing countries good deals on new coal-fired power plants.[7] China's decision to promote the sale of coal-fired power plants abroad as part of its Belt-and-Road initiative is facilitated by the fact that their emissions are considered irrelevant to China's Paris-Agreement performance. They are relevant to the recipient countries' performance, of course, but their *per capita* emissions – Pakistan's for example – are often still low beyond reproach. With expected lifespans of 30–40 years, these plants will add billions of tonnes of CO_2 to our atmosphere.

With these thoughts in mind, let us sketch a workable moral path to averting the looming climate catastrophe. We start with the scientific-community consensus that, to have a decent chance of success, we must prevent the Earth's average surface temperature from ever exceeding the pre-industrial level by more than 2 degrees Celsius. Doing so requires substantial cuts in greenhouse gas emissions. A plausible way of sharing the burdens of these cuts fairly among the generations envisions a glide path that reduces emissions by an equal percentage each year. Current data and predictive models suggest that the steepness of this glide path needs to be about 5% *per annum*. Humanity would then reduce anthropogenic CO_2 emissions form 43,000 Mt in 2019 to 30,000 in 2026, 20,000 in 2034, 12,000 in 2044 and 5000 in 2061.[8]

States are best positioned to specify and implement this constraint in an efficient and effective manner, through appropriate taxes on emissions, for example. So, it makes sense to distribute the task to them on a *per capita* basis. Because the human population is still increasing at about 1% annually, the required annual reduction in CO_2 emissions *per capita* must be set at approximately 6%. The uniform glide path for all states would start, then, with the 2019 level of 5.5 tonnes per year and person, and reduce from there to about 3 tonnes in 2029 and 1 tonne in 2047. This basic idea can readily be extended to include the full range of greenhouse gases.

Affluent countries greatly exceed the 5.5-tonne-*per-capita* ceiling. Saudi Arabia and the United Arab Emirates emit around 20 tonnes *per capita*, Australia, Canada and the US around 16, Japan 10, China 8, the EU 7.[9] These super-polluting countries bear the main burden of emission reduction. This seems fair on a principle of equality: no people can plausibly claim more extensive rights to pollute our planet than any other. It is generous, even, insofar as it leaves aside these countries' massive past emissions – and their massive wealth, created in emitting ways.

Affluent countries cannot reduce their emissions below the ceiling overnight. They should therefore, have an alternative option that ensures that the world as a whole complies with the glide path. The basic idea is obvious: affluent countries may approach the uniform glide path progressively, provided they make up for their remaining deficit by facilitating offsetting emissions reductions in other countries that are below that glide path.[10] For example, unable to reduce its CO_2 emissions to the global *per capita* ceiling immediately, Japan has the alternative option to reduce its emissions partway and then to achieve the remaining emissions reduction by helping one or more poorer countries install or switch to greener technologies. Countries can choose among potential partners and will tend to pursue the most cost-effective opportunities. Had such a scheme been in place, we would not have hundreds of coal-fired power plants under construction or in planning today. Instead, countries above the uniform glide path would volunteer to 'pay the difference' so that poorer countries have the electricity they need for their development – from renewable sources, at no extra cost to them.

2.3. The Oslo Principles

The arrangement just sketched follows the main outlines of the Oslo Principles formulated by the Expert Group on Global Climate Obligations.[11] Consisting mostly of lawyers, this group spent years exploring what legal duties states have in regard to the looming climate catastrophe, even apart from any explicit treaties or agreements they might enter, for example in the context of their UNFCCC negotiations. That there are such legal duties seems undeniable, given that a climate catastrophe would lead to violations of human rights on a horrendous scale. Clearly, states are not legally permitted to destroy with their emissions the preconditions of life on this planet. But what does this entail for the legal duties of any particular state? Cannot each of them say that its emissions would do no harm if other states appropriately curtailed theirs?

In response to this challenge, the expert group formulated the Oslo Principle as the – in its judgment – best reconstruction of existing law: of recognized human rights and other parts of international law, environmental law, tort law and private law. As such a reconstruction, the Oslo Principles have been an inspiration for important legal cases, most notably the celebrated *State of the Netherlands v. Urgenda Foundation*, first decided in 2015 and reaffirmed by the Netherlands Supreme Court in 2019.[12]

2.4. A global climate treaty

Even if progress is possible through legal suits in dozens of countries, it is preferable that states agree on something like the Oslo Principles and then start implementing it. This is what we here propose.

Such an Agreement would go beyond Paris in three main ways. First, states would all be judged by the same rules rather than each against its own self-chosen 'intended nationally determined contributions'. Second, this Agreement would involve the recognition of legally binding duties, rather than mere expressions of intent that states can ignore without penalty. Third, the Agreement would focus attention on the Global South, whose development we must green for any decent chance of saving our planet.

Nigeria's current CO_2 emissions are about 0.5 tonnes per person, apparently negligible. But in fact, Nigeria's decisions about how to grow its energy, cement, steel, agriculture and traffic sectors are of enormous importance. Nigeria has 210 million people now, and is projected to have 750 million by 2100. Its annual *per-capita* electricity consumption is 126 kWh now, only 1% of the US. How Nigeria and the other 150 countries of the Global South will develop themselves matters immensely. Our proposal would make these countries sought-after partners with whom richer countries must cooperate to compensate their delayed compliance with the – continuously declining – emissions ceiling.

Industrialized countries should reduce their emissions. But they can do vastly more for the world's climate through intelligent collaboration with developing countries. Our proposal makes good use of this fact. It would create a partnership market with below-ceiling countries on one side and above-ceiling countries on the other. Each state could negotiate with multiple potential partners on the other side, exploring alternative ideas and terms of collaboration, then make its choices from a position of equality. This would result in early uptake of advanced green technologies even in the poorest countries and a strong tendency toward the most cost-effective emissions reductions.

3. Promoting a global tax system that lessens inequality

The reforms proposed above should be complemented by reform of the international tax architecture which allows many of today's inequities to compound over time. The global pandemic has already bloated public spending and debt to sustain health care and employment. These costs must eventually be covered from tax revenues.

Flaws in the international tax architecture plainly aggravate inequalities and systematically undermine human rights, especially women's rights. For decades, the countries dominating the OECD have set the rules for international tax and financial transparency. Under these rules, tax minimization strategies by multinational companies (MNCs) are not marginal activities, but central to their global operations. All serious estimates, by UNCTAD, the IMF and Tax Justice Network, show that the costs of tax abuse are proportionally higher for lower-income countries.[13]

Keeping these realities in mind, we support six major global tax reforms for the post-pandemic world.

3.1. Eliminate fossil-fuel subsidies

In 2015, the IMF published a famous report showing that fossil-fuel subsidies around the world amounted to some \$5.3 trillion *per annum* (Coady et al., 2015), including the cost of negative externalities, such as clean-up and health-related costs, that fossil-fuel burning imposes upon governments and taxpayers.[14] These subsidies should be phased out, ensuring that users of fossil-fuel-derived energy bear the full cost of their consumption. This phase-out would raise the cost of such energy; but any resulting hardships could be averted or mitigated by distributing some of the additional revenues collected or retained by governments. For example, were the US to add \$1 in new taxes on each gallon of gasoline or diesel fuel sold, it could spend half of the additional \$190 billion raised on annual \$1900-per-person payments to the poorest 100 million US residents.[15] This way, poor households would not be hurt but would still have the same incentives as others to reduce their fossil-fuel consumption. The key gains from the subsidy phase-out would be to level the playing field among diverse energy sources and to ensure that energy consumers have appropriate incentives that reflect their consumption's true full cost, including to future generations.

3.2. Stem the abuse of tax havens through a global minimum tax

Among the historic post-colonial tragedies developing countries had to face is abuse of tax havens. MNCs routinely use them in their international tax planning strategies, creating subsidiaries in low-tax jurisdictions where profits earned globally can conveniently be parked. By housing patents, copyrights, and other intellectual property, and through transfer mispricing, these subsidiaries divert income from other, developing and developed countries, which suffer substantial tax revenue losses as a result.

According to the IMF, tax havens collectively cost governments $500–600 billion annually in lost corporate taxes (Cobham & Jansky, 2018; Crivelli et al., 2016). Low- and lower-middle-income countries suffer grossly disproportional shares of this loss with devastating impact on their populations: each year, they lose $200 billion or 17.5% of their tax revenues, substantially more than the $150 billion they receive in development assistance.

Were there a minimum tax applied to all tax haven subsidiaries at a rate comparable to the marginal tax rates applicable in the MNCs' home jurisdictions, then incentives to shift profits into tax havens would be much reduced. This would benefit developed and developing countries and correct a major flaw of the global financial architecture.

The 2017 Tax Act in the United States created such a minimum tax, the Global Intangible Low-Taxed Income (GILTI) tax, to weaken financial incentives for US-based MNCs to shift income to low- or no-tax jurisdictions. We additionally propose doubling the GILTI tax from the current 10.5% to 21%, which is the corporate tax rate inaugurated in the 2017 legislation, which might then become the global standard. If all OECD countries followed such a standard, tax haven abuse would gradually disappear. This could be the start of a 'New Deal' advancing tax justice worldwide.

3.3. Reduce the risk of recessions globally by reinstituting Glass–Steagall

The global economy was hit hard by the 2008–2009 recession, which was largely driven by deregulation in the financial service sector and the 1999 repeal of the Glass–Steagall Act, separating commercial from investment banking. Banks' speculative activities in subprime mortgage securities threatened to precipitate another great depression. This was narrowly averted through the Emergency Economic Stabilization Act of 2008, which created the $700-billion Troubled Asset Relief Program to purchase toxic assets from banks. Had Glass–Steagall still been in place, this huge bailout would have been avoided.

The fundamental issue is whether financial institutions should be free to speculate under rules that allow them to profit from any gains while imposing risks of catastrophic loss upon the public. When taking office in 1933, Franklin Roosevelt strongly warned against such asymmetric risk assignment: 'We do not wish to make the United States Government liable for the mistakes and errors of individual banks, and put a premium on unsound banking in the future'.[16] This set the stage for the Glass–Steagall Act, Federal Deposit Insurance, and other New Deal provisions.

It is ironic that another Democratic president, Bill Clinton, got Glass–Steagall repealed 66 years later. In the aftermath of the 2008–2009 recession, yet another Democratic President, Barack Obama, in 2010 signed into law the Wall Street Reform and Consumer Protection Act ('Dodd–Frank'), which included the Volcker Rule barring banks from certain speculative investments. But since then many of Dodd–Frank's regulatory provisions, including the Volcker Rule, have been substantially diluted or rolled back. This puts the global economy at risk once again through unstable markets and widespread speculation by Wall Street, increasing the likelihood of recessions, depressions, and rampant unemployment as witnessed in the current pandemic.

Protections of the public against speculative excesses in the financial sector should be reinstituted – urgently so in view of the resource constraints imposed by the ongoing pandemic. Here the US, the world's largest economy, should set an example and encourage other states to follow suit. The needed reforms are feasible, as it is now widely understood that financial-sector regulation is necessary if capitalism is to be stable and to serve the interests of all. Without such reforms, the risk of future recessions and depressions will always hang over the global economy like a sword of Damocles.

3.4. Implement a financial transactions tax globally

A tax on trades of financial assets has important advantages. It would dampen some financial activity and help reshape a political economy in which finance has become overly dominant. Primarily affecting wealthy individuals and large corporations, such a financial transaction tax (FTT) would be progressive, thus moderating inequality. It could generate substantial revenues, much needed by governments in these perilous times. These advantages would give the FTT broad appeal as would the perception that the rich and the financial sector have not been contributing their fair share to the costs of government.

An early FTT proponent was Nobel laureate James Tobin who, starting in the early 1970s, proposed a tax on currency transactions to reduce speculation-induced exchange rate fluctuations and thereby to enable national governments and central banks better to adapt their monetary policies to domestic economic conditions. Set at 0.5%, as he envisioned in the 1990s (Tobin, 1994), his tax would also raise substantial revenues. Presently the *daily* volume of worldwide currency transactions is an incredible $6.6 trillion.[17] Even if a Tobin Tax achieved its purpose by reducing this volume dramatically, say by a factor of 10, it would still raise over $800 billion annually.[18]

Parallel reasoning applies to markets in virtual currencies, stocks, bonds, commodities, futures, options, swaps and other derivatives.[19] All these markets are subject to speculation-fueled instability – through computer-driven high-frequency trading, for instance – which even a tiny FTT would reduce substantially. How much revenue such a tax would raise depends on its rate and on how severely it would, as intended, dampen financial activity. The details would need to be worked out on the basis of empirical studies and international negotiations.

In view of the widespread persistence of severe deprivations among the world's poor, which our governments with their Sustainable Development Goals Agenda have yet once more promised to eradicate, in view of the enormous restructuring investments needed for a fast and adequate response to the ongoing climate emergency, and in view of the massive revenue needs generated by the COVID-19 pandemic and its foreseeable aftermath, a well-structured, internationally coordinated FTT is urgently needed. That such a tax would also curb the excesses of the financial sector, stabilize financial markets and reduce socio-economic inequality around the world are additional important advantages. The present time presents a rare opportunity to overcome the strong lobbying pressure of the financial sector by instituting such a broad FTT.

3.5. Ensure fair value for natural resource sales

The mineral resources of poorer countries can play a crucial role in their development. Yet, all-too-often this finite wealth is siphoned off by foreign-owned MNCs, which carry out most large-scale mining operations. One favourite method involves so-called tax expenditures, special tax exemptions or reductions, commonly justified as necessary inducements to attract foreign investment, but often heavily lobbied for by their recipients or even bought through bribes and other favours to officials. Another usual method of tax avoidance is profit shifting into tax havens through artificial and mispriced transactions between local subsidiaries of an MNC and other subsidiaries that the same MNC creates in tax havens. Such related-party transactions offer ample opportunities for tax avoidance by under-invoicing exported minerals and over-invoicing imported goods and services. A major share of developing countries' $200-billion tax loss comes from the mining sector, lending credibility to the adage that colonialism never ended but merely changed business plans.

Tax cheating by MNCs impedes development also by undermining the competitiveness of local firms, which lack similar tax dodging opportunities. Further harm to development is done when importing countries strongly encourage – through staggered tariffs, for instance – the exportation of raw materials in their rawest form, so as to ensure that value-adding processing happens in their own countries. These enormously harmful practices are made harder to overcome by the great asymmetry in expertise and power between developing country officials, on the one hand, and representatives of large MNCs and affluent countries, on the other. Very rarely do African tax officials have the expertise, time and training to thoroughly analyse a hugely complex web of inter-related corporations and their internal transactions – and in those few cases, a lucrative job offer can most likely induce the officials to switch sides. Similarly, state officials and legislators are easily influenced through political contributions, gifts or bribes to support arrangements that favour foreigners over their own country and its people.

Reform is needed on three levels. First, developing countries should jointly propose changes to unfair international rules and practices, most plausibly perhaps through the United Nations Conference on Trade and Development, the International Monetary Fund or the International Commission for the Reform of Corporate Taxation. Such international rules should require firms to adopt principles on responsible tax: making boards accountable for tax policy, being transparent about subsidiaries owned around the world, and publishing a tax strategy that is clear to all stakeholders. Second, developing countries should take parallel policy action in concert, thereby reducing opportunities for MNCs and governments to play them off against one another. Third, developing countries should act unilaterally to better protect themselves against MNC predations, for example by hiring and training first-rate tax administrators, as supported by Tax Inspectors Without Borders, a joint OECD-UNDP initiative.

3.6. Place a fair progressive tax on internationally operating digital firms

The post-pandemic world is seeing acceleration of a long-standing trend toward digital businesses, defined as ones that use technology and artificial intelligence to create new value in business models and customer experience, including cloud storage, digital shopping, and educational services such as Zoom and Google Meet.

Depending on one's definition, the digital economy is now worth between $4 and $14 trillion annually, accounting for well over half of all service exports (UN, 2021, p. 10). This economic sector is highly profitable and reaches across international borders even without a physical presence abroad. Taxing this sector is challenging, and traditional ways of measuring profitability and allocating profits among jurisdictions prove inadequate.

For a sustainable economic recovery, governments need to implement a more progressive digital services tax, to capture in a fair and equitable manner some of the economic rents that digital MNCs capture in the countries where they market their services. Currently, these MNCs enjoy the best of both worlds: surging profits in most markets while avoiding equitable taxation thanks to an outdated tax system.

Once more we favour taxing MNCs as unitary firms. Profits should be allocated among jurisdictions on the basis of factors that are easily quantifiable, reflect real activities, and balance supply and demand. These factors are employees, physical assets, and sales. Only such an approach can ensure that attributed income and taxes paid are proportionate to the MNC's actual economic activity in each jurisdiction.

In its important public comment on this issue, the International Commission for the Reform of Corporate Taxation states:

> The allocation of multinationals' profits between jurisdictions for taxation purposes is a fundamentally distributive task; revisions to the rules will result in redistribution of taxing rights, and this should take into account the impact on both developed and developing countries, their relative contribution to the global economy and their fiscal needs. (ICRICT, 2019, p. 6)

For the sake of developing countries especially, taxation of digital income should be fair, formula-based, and not subject to manipulation that benefits the large MNCs providing such services. This issue is currently under negotiation, and we urge agreement on a formulary-based system as outlined above.

4. Conclusion

Our present challenge is not merely to cope with a global pandemic, but also to address comprehensively the serious vulnerabilities and inequities it has exposed. As in the 1930s, when the New Deal reforms were implemented, the crisis we face is a rare opportunity to institute bold structural reforms that can revive and sustain prosperity in the post-Covid-19 world. We must not waste this opportunity.

We have argued for three reform agendas that might plausibly emerge from the present COVID-19 crisis. These reforms are complementary in various ways; for example, the reforms proposed in Section 3 could provide some of the funds needed for the reforms advocated in the first two sections. These reforms are also strategic by bringing further important reforms within reach.

Transformative and yet realistic, these reforms are now feasible if we can mobilize sufficient international support for them. Doing so is not easy. But a return to business as usual would be far worse, certainly for the poor and for people with a conscience.

Notes

1. https://www.who.int/neglected_diseases/diseases/en/.
2. https://www.who.int/tb/en/, https://www.who.int/malaria/en/.
3. The Clinton Health Access Initiative found that, four years after its introduction, only about 7% of the 71 million persons living with hepatitis C have been treated. The other 66 million remain ill and continue to spread the disease (CHAI, 2020, p. 8).
4. Proven reserves of crude oil alone are worth around $100 trillion, more than the current annual gross world product.
5. In 1835, Great Britain borrowed the present equivalent of about $300 billion to compensate some 3000 slaveholders for their lost 'property' – the slaves of course got nothing. Repayment of this huge loan took until 2015. https://www.theguardian.com/news/2018/mar/29/slavery-abolition-compensation-when-will-britain-face-up-to-its-crimes-against-humanity and https://www.independent.co.uk/news/uk/home-news/britains-colonial-shame-slave-owners-given-huge-payouts-after-abolition-8508358.html.
6. https://www.worldometers.info/coal/coal-consumption-by-country.
7. https://phys.org/news/2020-12-china-foreign-coal-global-climate.html. China is not alone. Since the Paris Agreement, the 60 largest commercial and investment banks, led by JPMorgan Chase, Citi and Bank of America, have collectively provided $3.8 trillion in financing to fossil-fuel companies. https://www.cnbc.com/2021/03/24/how-much-the-largest-banks-have-invested-in-fossil-fuel-report.html.
8. https://www.statista.com/statistics/276629/global-co2-emissions/.
9. https://en.wikipedia.org/wiki/List_of_countries_by_carbon_dioxide_emissions.
10. A similar idea underlay the Clean Development Mechanism under the Kyoto Protocol, though its implementation was deeply flawed. https://en.wikipedia.org/wiki/Clean_Development_Mechanism.

11. https://globaljustice.yale.edu/oslo-principles-global-climate-change-obligations.
12. https://www.urgenda.nl/en/themas/climate-case/global-climate-litigation/, https://en.wikipedia.org/wiki/State_of_the_Netherlands_v._Urgenda_Foundation.
13. http://taxjustice.wpengine.com/wp-content/uploads/2017/11/Tax-dodging-the-scale-of-the-problem-TJN-Briefing.pdf.
14. In 2015, the largest subsidizers were China, the US and Russia, with $1400, $649 and $551 billion, respectively. https://www.eesi.org/papers/view/fact-sheet-fossil-fuel-subsidies-a-closer-look-at-tax-breaks-and-societal-costs.
15. Of course, such a scheme could work elsewhere as well: in China, Europe, Latin America, the Arab world and Australia, where such 'carbon pricing', introduced by the Labour Party under Julia Gillard, was in effect 2012–2014 before being revoked after an election win by the Liberal Party under Tony Abbott. https://en.wikipedia.org/wiki/Carbon_pricing_in_Australia.
16. https://en.wikipedia.org/wiki/Presidency_of_Franklin_D._Roosevelt,_first_and_second_terms.
17. https://www.bloomberg.com/news/articles/2019-09-16/global-currency-trading-surges-to-6-6-trillion-a-day-market.
18. Assuming 250 trading days, $6,600,000,000 * 250 * 0.5% / 10. This revenue would be diminished somewhat by the cost of administration and enforcement.
19. Interestingly, New York State has had an FTT for stock transactions since 1906, but has chosen, since 1981, fully to rebate this tax. https://www.vox.com/2014/11/20/7254003/financial-transaction-tax. The rate ranges from $0.0125 to $0.05 per share, depending on the share price.

Disclosure statement

No potential conflict of interest was reported by the authors.

ORCID

Thomas Pogge ⓘ http://orcid.org/0000-0001-9081-1314

References

CHAI. (2020). *Hepatitis C market report, Clinton health access initiative.* https://3cdmh310dov3470e6x160esb-wpengine.netdna-ssl.com/wp-content/uploads/2020/05/Hepatitis-C-Market-Report_Issue-1_Web.pdf
Coady, D., Parry, I., Sears, L., & Shang, B. (2015). *How large are global energy subsidies?* (IMF Working Paper 15/105). https://www.imf.org/external/pubs/ft/wp/2015/wp15105.pdf

Cobham, A., & Jansky, P. (2018). Global distribution of revenue loss from corporate tax avoidance: Re-estimation and country results. *Journal of International Development, 30*(2), 206–232. https://doi.org/10.1002/jid.3348

Crivelli, E., de Mooij, R., & Keen, M. (2016). Base erosion, profit shifting and developing countries. *FinanzArchiv: Public Finance Analysis, 72*(3), 268–301. https://www.imf.org/en/Publications/WP/Issues/2016/12/31/Base-Erosion-Profit-Shifting-and-Developing-Countries-42973

ICRICT. (2019). *International corporate tax reform: Towards a fair and comprehensive solution.* Independent Commission for the Reform of International Corporate Taxation. https://www.icrict.com/press-release/2019/10/6/icrict-report-current-reform-of-international-tax-system-radical-change-or-yet-another-short-term-fix

IFPMA. (2017). *The pharmaceutical industry and global health.* International Federation of Pharmaceutical Manufacturers & Associations. https://www.ifpma.org/resource-centre/ifpma-facts-and-figures-report

Nocera, J. (2018, November 27). Wall Street wants the best patents, not the best drugs. *Bloombergquint.* https://www.bloombergquint.com/view/gilead-s-cures-for-hepatitis-c-were-not-a-great-business-model

Pogge, T. (2010). Poverty, climate change and overpopulation. *Georgia Journal of International and Comparative Law, 38*(3), 525–542.

Sachs, J. (2015, April 18). The drug that is bankrupting America. *Huffington Post.* https://www.huffpost.com/entry/the-drug-that-is-bankrupt_b_6692340

Tobin, J. (1994). A tax on international currency transactions. In United Nations Development Program, *Human development report* (p. 70). Oxford University Press.

UN. (2021). *COVID-19 and e-commerce: A global review.* https://unctad.org/system/files/official-document/dtlstict2020d13_en_0.pdf

The post-pandemic world and the prospect for global justice: a commentary

Habibul Haque Khondker ⓘ

ABSTRACT

The pandemic has wiped out over 4 million human lives and caused huge economic loss. As poverty forecasts famine, the super-rich became richer. The consequence of the pandemic has also shrunk the democratic space. In selected cases, the growing perception of social inequality matched the number of caseloads of infections and deaths. The response to the pandemic varied depending not only on the effectiveness of the responses by the respective governments but also by the presence of scientific thinking in society. The pandemic and the distribution of vaccine highlighted the need for interdependence and cooperation between the nations. It has also created a need for renewing global justice based on humanity and rationality in the post-pandemic world.

By the third week of July 2021, loss of lives due to Covid-19 reached 4.1 million worldwide (and counting), with countless livelihoods imperilled by the measures designed to combat the pandemic, and the pandemic rolled back decades of achievements in poverty reduction globally. The United Nations predicts COVID-19 will slash $8.5 trillion from the world economy over the next two years and would push 34 million people to extreme poverty (UNDESA, 2020). The IMF estimated that close to 95 million people are under the threshold of extreme poverty in 2020 (IMF, 2021). The Oxfam report of 2021 painted a gloomier picture showing a sharp increase in global income inequality, and estimated that the total number of people living in poverty could have increased between 200 and 500 million. By the third week of June, the World Food Programme declared that 41 million people were facing famine (WFP, 2021). The fortune of the billionaires rose by 27% during the pandemic.

Worldwide, while poverty and hunger increased, billionaires' wealth increased by a staggering $3.9 trillion between 18 March and 31 December 2020, according to Oxfam. The world's 10 richest billionaires have collectively seen their wealth increase by $540bn over this period (OXFAM, 2021). The wealth increase of the 10 richest men during the pandemic was enough to buy vaccines for all (Read, 2020). As poor people became poorer, the number of millionaires increased by 5.2 million to 56.1 million globally, according to a Credit Suisse research (BBC, 2021). This is one of the most telling paradoxes of the impact of the pandemic. A major disruptor in history, the pandemic, has accentuated the pre-existing poverty and inequality of the world.

Arundhati Roy views the pandemic as a portal, and wrote: 'Historically, pandemics have forced humans to break with the past and imagine their world anew. This one is no different. It is a portal, a gateway between one world and the next' (Roy, 2020). Henry Kissinger (2020) also opined that the post-pandemic world will change forever. Clearly, changes in schooling, business and work that began prior to pandemic will be accelerated, but only time will tell how many structural changes can be realistically expected in the post-pandemic world. The pandemic has revealed the glaring ills of the twenty-first-century capitalist world economy for what it is, unequal and unjust. But, it has provided an occasion for tightening the grip of political control and reducing democratic space.

Even during the thick pandemic, the world has witnessed race riots, wars, land-grabs and dispossessions. The ills of the world were outdone by the news of the pandemic in the media, but they never receded for long. Pandemics in the fourteenth century have shaped society, paving the way for the end of feudalism. However, such far historical parallels may be unrealistic. The pandemic provided an excuse for authoritarian regimes to be more authoritarian, pushing away the few gains for democracy here and there. In 2020, the number of 'free' countries in the world, according to the Freedom House Report, got drastically reduced since the beginning of decline of democracy 15 years ago. Conversely, the number of 'not free' countries got highly increased (Repucci & Slipowitz, 2021). Advanced surveillance technology at one level was used effectively in contact tracing to help curb the spread of coronavirus, yet at another level it encroached on the privacy of the citizens.

The spread of social inequality and the reaction to it have been uneven worldwide. A Pew survey revealed that because of the pandemic, sentiments of social division, presumably class division, have risen in the Global North. However, interestingly the negative sentiments vary from 88% in the USA, 83% in the Netherlands, 77% in Germany and Spain on the one hand and New Zealand, 23%, Taiwan, 20% and Singapore 12% on the other. These numbers are positively related to caseloads and mortality (Devlin et al., 2021). The efficacy of the states in dealing with the pandemic crisis impacts the perceptions of social fissures. Death rates per million people varied significantly. Compare deaths per million of the USA (1,862), Germany (1,728), Spain (1,087), The Netherlands (1,033), on the one hand, and Singapore (6), and New Zealand (5)[1] on the other.

The Covid-19 pandemic has been a moving target. The survey results provide only a snapshot. Countries that did well in containing the pandemic early, such as Australia, lagged behind in the rolling out of vaccines. For several countries – both market-based liberal democracies in Europe and coordinated capitalist societies – were on a backfoot as the crisis seemed to be intractable. At the time of writing (July 2021), half of Australia is under hard lockdown, Spain, Italy and Portugal are open for business-attracting tourists, and England seems to have left the worst behind by removing nearly all the restrictions by the third week of July 2021. Based on the rate of death per million, New Zealand may be identified as the best performer in managing the crisis. The response to the Covid-19 pandemic in China as well as in the Tiger economies, Hong Kong, Taiwan, and Singapore highlighted the importance of the statist command and control approaches to crisis management. The role and relevance of state capacity has returned to both public and academic discussions to the dismay of free-market thinkers. State capacity and social trust with quality of political leadership have been advanced as explanations for the successful handling of the crisis (Fukuyama & Lopez-Calva, 2021). Several writers examined the issues of governance, by focusing on the role of state in handling the Covid-19 crisis. The state response, ranging from Africa, Europe to East Asia and Latin America, showed variations and specificities that defied patterns and models and are the results of a confluence of variables (Nederveen Pieterse, 2021). While it showed the importance of the state rather than the market, it led to the shrinking space of democracy with implications for the post-Covid world.

Comparative studies also brought to light the presence of rational thinking, as revealed in the acceptance of science, scientific evidence, and policies guided by science in a society, as a key variable. Governance does not occur in a vacuum. Apart from the efficacy of the institutions of society, one needs to consider whether the behaviour and particularly actions of the people are guided by scientific facts or not. In a joint study by scholars at Harvard and Cornell, Covid-19 responses across 18 countries were examined (Jasanoff et al., 2021). In terms of responses and the effectiveness of responses, countries have been classified as Control, Consensus, and Chaos countries. China is a control country, so is Singapore. Germany approximates a consensus country. Brazil, Italy, USA and India are chaos countries. How scientific is the culture of a given society? How strong, if at all, is public reason in that society? It boils down to how gullible are the people to alternative assumptions, that is to non-scientific or pseudoscientific beliefs? The discussion of the importance of science and its various applications in society and the social and political factors in the use of science and broadly scientific rationality, will remain another point of contention in the post-pandemic world.

OECD projects a global economic growth of 5.8% for 2021 (OECD, 2021). Some countries are poised to recover faster than the others. A robust projected growth of the US economy hides uneven effects of the pandemic globally. China managed the crisis better than most through the hammer and dance strategy (surely, more hammer at the early stage than dance). A group of economists at Toulouse School of Economics in France in mid-May 2020 introduced these useful metaphors in recommending a nuanced response to the pandemic crisis, addressing both the economic and health policy objectives. The coming of the new administration in the USA changed the distribution of vaccine from a Trumpian dismal and denial approach reaching nearly 340 million vaccines (102 per 100) by the third week of July 2021 (New York Times, 2021). The USA, once a chaos country under Mr. Trump, has come out of that label under President Biden. The link between increased vaccination, recovery, and economic growth is unsurprising.

The important lesson, to learn from the Covid-19 pandemic, is that there is no substitute for global cooperation and global solidarity in handling catastrophes like a pandemic. The sharing of the DNA sequencing of the virus and the protocols of treatment were promising in containing the epidemic, though cooperation somewhat stalled in the sharing of vaccines. The lessons of cooperation need to be extended to focus on the ecological balance and sustainability at the global scale. The extreme weather disasters ranging from drought in the Northwest America and the heavy rain-induced flooding in parts of Germany, Belgium, and Holland and China in the summer of 2021 are signs of climate change, which need to be addressed globally.

As vaccines developed in record time provided a glimmer of hope, new strains of the virus – Delta, Delta-2, Lambda – appeared, and the light at the end of the proverbial tunnel began to dim again. The sluggish distribution of the vaccine revealed deeper politics at the global and local levels. *The Guardian* sounds an alarm as most of the poor countries of the world are unable to buy vaccines from the large pharmaceutical companies. The emergence of Delta-2 virus, which caused a surge of deaths in India, has delayed the export of vaccines to the poor countries (The Guardian, 2021). As of 23 July 2021, 26.9% of the world population has received at least one vaccine dose. For the Global South the figure is only 1.1% (Ourworldindata, 2021). In the distribution of vaccines globally, China is stepping into a position of leadership, and Covid-19 may accelerate China's ascendance as a superpower (BBC, 2020).

It is now increasingly obvious that the Covid-19 pandemic can only be addressed by global cooperation. A lot depends on the political will of world leaders, who must cooperate in resolving the global issues of global warming and the growing social inequality. There is an increasing need to be more vocal and public-spirited and to renew the call for global justice and to forge solidarity and promote public education, urging people to think broadly about overcoming structural racism, demanding equal rights, and climate justice. In an interconnected world, a pandemic anywhere is a pandemic everywhere. In a similar vein, a solution everywhere should be the priority for solution anywhere. The need of the hour is to vote for more globalism and global – albeit, critical – cosmopolitanism (Gills et al., 2017). Kissinger (2020) reminded of the responsibility of states for ensuring 'security, order, economic well-being, and justice'. The challenge is to enlarge the scope of this from the state to the supra-state, i.e. the global level. The problem at heart is the problem of a lack of an equitable world and absence of justice. A call for global justice, based on a shared belief in rationality and common humanity, is the need for the post-pandemic world.

Note

1. Data as of 30 June 2021 (Worldometers).

Disclosure statement

No potential conflict of interest was reported by the author(s).

ORCID

Habibul Haque Khondker ⓘ http://orcid.org/0000-0002-5545-7599

References

BBC. (2020). Chinese economy to overtake us 'by 2028' due to Covid. https://www.bbc.com/news/world-asia-china-55454146

BBC. (2021, June 23). BBC News. https://www.bbc.com/news/business-57575077

Devlin, K., Fagan, M., & Connaughton, A. (2021). People in Advanced Economies Say Their Society is More Divided Than Before Pandemic. Pew Survey. https://www.pewresearch.org/global/2021/06/23/people-in-advanced-economies-say-their-society-is-more-divided-than-before-pandemic/?utm_source=Eurasia+Group+Signal&utm_campaign=8564bd39ca-EMAIL_CAMPAIGN_2021_06_25_10_47&utm_medium=email&utm_term=0_e605619869-8564bd39ca-170469526

Fukuyama, F., & Lopez-Calva, L. F. (2021, June 24). Pandemic and political performance. *Project Syndicate.* https://www.project-syndicate.org/commentary/pandemic-political-decay-latin-america-caribbean-by-francis-fukuyama-and-luis-felipe-lopez-calva-2021-06

Gills, B. K., Hosseini, S. A. H., & Goodman, J. (2017). Theorizing alternatives to capital: Towards a critical cosmopolitanist framework. *European Journal of Social Theory, 20*(4), 437–454. https://doi.org/10.1177/1368431016642609

The Guardian. (2021). Covid vaccines: Indian export delay deals blow to poor countries. https://www.theguardian.com/world/2021/may/19/poorer-countries-face-long-delays-receiving-covid-vaccines

IMF. (2021). World economic outlook: Managing divergent recoveries. https://www.imf.org/en/Publications/WEO/Issues/2021/03/23/world-economic-outlook-april-2021

Jasanoff, S., Hilgartner, S., Hurlbut, J. B., Ozgode, O., & Rayzberg, M. (2021). *Comparative covid response: Crisis, knowledge, politics: Interim report, J. F. Kennedy school.* Harvard University.

Kissinger, H. (2020, April 3). The Coronovirus pandemic will forever alter the world. *Wall Street Journal.* https://www.wsj.com/articles/the-coronavirus-pandemic-will-forever-alter-the-world-order-11585953005

Nederveen Pieterse, J. (2021). Introduction. In J. Nederveen Pieterse, H. Lim, & H. Khondker (Eds.), *Covid-19 and governance* (pp. 1–11). Routledge.

New York Times. (2021). Covid world vaccination tracker. https://www.nytimes.com/interactive/2021/world/covid-vaccinations-tracker.html

OECD. (2021). https://www.oecd.org/economic-outlook/

Ourworldindata. (2021). https://ourworldindata.org/covid-vaccinations

OXFAM. (2021). https://oxfamilibrary.openrepository.com/bitstream/handle/10546/621149/bp-the-inequality-virus-250121-en.pdf

Read, S. (2020, October 7). Billionaires see fortunes rise by 27% during the pandemic. https://www.bbc.com/news/business-54446285

Repucci, S., & Slipowitz, A. (2021). Freedom in the world 2021: Democracy under siege. Freedom House. https://freedomhouse.org/report/freedom-world/2021/democracy-under-siege

Roy, A. (2020). The pandemic is a portal. *Financial Times*, April 3. https://www.ft.com/content/10d8f5e8-74eb-11ea-95fe-fcd274e920ca

UNDESA. (2020). https://www.un.org/en/desa/covid-19-slash-global-economic-output-85-trillion-over-next-two-years

World Food Program. (2021). https://www.wfp.org/news/wfp-says-41-million-people-now-imminent-risk-famine-without-urgent-funding-and-immediate

Worldometers. (2021, June 30). https://www.worldometers.info/coronavirus/

Index

Note: Figures are indicated by *italics*.

For Product Safety Concerns and Information please contact our EU
representative GPSR@taylorandfrancis.com
Taylor & Francis Verlag GmbH, Kaufingerstraße 24, 80331 München, Germany

www.ingramcontent.com/pod-product-compliance
Lightning Source LLC
Chambersburg PA
CBHW081537220326
41598CB00036B/6460